ACTA UNIVERSITATIS UPSALIENSIS

Studies in Bioethics and Research Ethics

4

Anders Nordgren (ed.)

Gene Therapy and Ethics

UPPSALA 1999

ABSTRACT

Nordgren, A. (ed.), 1998. Gene Therapy and Ethics. Acta Universitatis Upsaliensis. *Studies in Bioethics and Research Ethics 4*. 175 pp. Uppsala. ISBN 91-554-4640-X.

Gene therapy is a set of approaches to the treatment of human disease based on transfer of genetic material (DNA) into an individual. In 1990, the first officially authorized experiment of gene therapy was performed. At present, several hundred patients have participated in trials all over the world. Many scientists maintain that gene therapy has an extraordinary potential in the long term for the treatment of human diseases, although clinical efficacy has not yet been definitely demonstrated.

However, gene therapy research and its clinical application raises many ethical, legal, and social questions. In order to give an opportunity for geneticists, bioethicists, social scientists and others to discuss these issues, the Centre for Research Ethics at Uppsala University and the Swedish University of Agricultural Sciences organized a conference in 1998. The conference was arranged in collaboration with the Department of Public Health and Caring Sciences in Uppsala and the Kennedy Institute of Ethics in Washington DC. Most of the lectures and contributions to the seminars at the conference are, with some revisions, collected in this volume. The aim of publication is to stimulate further discussion and research on the ethical, legal, and social implications of gene therapy.

Key words: gene therapy, gene transfer, genetic enhancement, somatic gene therapy, germ-line gene therapy, genetic engineering, bioethics, policy, social responsibility, eugenics.

Anders Nordgren, Department of Public Health and Caring Sciences (Biomedical Ethics), Uppsala Science Park, SE-751 85, Uppsala, Sweden.

ISSN 1402-3148
ISBN 91-554-4640-X

Typesetting: Editorial Office, Uppsala University
Printed in Sweden by Elandes Gotab, Stockholm 1999
Distributor: Uppsala University Library, Uppsala, Sweden

Contents

ANDERS NORDGREN

Introduction

Gene therapy is a set of approaches to the treatment of human disease based on transfer of genetic material (DNA) into an individual. In 1990, the first officially authorized experiment of gene therapy was performed. At present, several hundred patients have participated in trials all over the world. Many scientists maintain that gene therapy has an extraordinary potential in the long term for the treatment of human diseases, although clinical efficacy has not yet been definitely demonstrated.[1]

Gene therapy research and its application raises many ethical, legal and social questions. In order to give an opportunity for geneticists, bioethicists, social scientists and others to discuss these issues, the Centre for Research Ethics at Uppsala University and the Swedish University of Agricultural Sciences organized a conference in 1998. The conference was arranged in collaboration with the Department of Public Health and Caring Sciences in Uppsala and the Kennedy Institute of Ethics in Washington DC. Most of the lectures and contributions to the seminars are, with some revisions, collected in this volume. The aim of publication is to stimulate further discussion and research on the ethical, legal and social implications of gene therapy.

In order to help the reader to find his or her way through the volume, the contributions have been divided into five sections. Many of the papers could have been placed in more than one section. Below I shall give a preview of the key ideas of the different papers.

Internal and external perspectives

In all bioethical discussions, it is important to be aware of the perspectives of different categories of people. This holds for the discussion of gene therapy as well. Here it is useful to make a distinction between internal and external perspectives. The internal perspectives are those of the scientists working in the field. The external perspectives are those of the general public, ethicists, journalists, politicians, and others. Both kinds of perspectives are legitimate. Naturally, gene therapy researchers have a right to have their own view on what they are doing. But their research is a social activity which affects the society at large and this makes the external perspectives legitimate as well. Both kinds of perspectives are also necessary in order to give the development of the research an ethically acceptable direction. This requires a dialogue between people representing these different kinds of perspectives. However, as Charles Weiner stresses in his paper, if we look at earlier debates on genetic engineering, we become aware of the risk that ethics is never allowed to really influence the research. Technical matters and ethical matters are kept apart.

Gene therapy: some distinctions

When we discuss the ethical aspects of gene therapy, it is important to make a distinction between ethical issues raised by:

- gene therapy research, and
- gene therapy.

In the former case, special problems of research ethics are raised. In the latter case, social aspects of the use of gene therapy are central. In this volume, both the research and its possible application in society are discussed.

In an ethical discussion, it might also be important to make certain distinctions between different kinds of gene therapy. Several years ago LeRoy Walters suggested a classification that has become classical in the bioethics literature. He distinguished the following kinds of genetic modification:

(1) somatic gene therapy,
(2) germ-line gene therapy,
(3) somatic genetic enhancement, and
(4) germ-line genetic enhancement.[2]

Somatic gene therapy is presently the only kind that is tested by scientists, and it is not particularly disputed. The other kinds, however, are all very controversial.[3]

The four-fold classification is now being challenged. In his contribution to this volume, Walters himself says that while the line between interventions on somatic cells and on the germ-line is rather sharp and clear, the line between therapy and enhancement is not quite as distinct. The latter is also stressed by Eric Juengst in his paper. Should disease-related enhancement, e.g. improvement of the immune system from normal to above normal, be classified as enhancement or as therapy? However, the first mentioned distinction, the one between somatic gene therapy and germ-line gene therapy, is not completely clear, either. Somatic gene therapy might sometimes have unintended effects on the germ-line.

Recently, a supplement to the division has also been suggested. It has often been presupposed that genetic interventions are limited to the nuclear genome. Given recent advances in genetics, however, the mitochondrial genome and diseases must be considered as well. This adds a new dimension to both somatic gene therapy and germ-line gene therapy.[4]

It might be disputed whether all of the above mentioned distinctions are ethically relevant. But it is quite clear that they are useful to keep in mind in any debate on gene therapy and its ethical implications, at least in order to understand the debate as such. Most of the distinctions will be referred to in this book.

Science

In December 1995 a Panel appointed by the National Institutes of Health (NIH) in the United States came forward with the verdict that somatic gene therapy research had in fact not been as successful as many researchers had proclaimed. The Panel charged the scientists for "overselling" their research. No real breakthroughs had been seen. No clinical efficacy had been achieved.[5] The question therefore becomes: how far has gene therapy research come today?

In this volume, present-day somatic gene therapy research is presented by two important scientists. The first presentation is by Edvard Smith, a Swedish gene therapy researcher who works on genetic approaches to, for instance, immunodeficiency diseases. Smith briefly describes which diseases are potential targets for gene therapy, how gene therapy works, and which gene transfer techniques are available today. He is confident that in the future it is likely that gene therapy will develop into an efficient tool with few side effects.

The second description of the scientific aspects of gene therapy is given by Malcolm Brenner. Brenner is one of the leading researchers on gene therapy in the world today. He develops cell and gene therapies for catastrophic diseases in children. Brenner concludes that while the results of gene therapy for non-malignant conditions have been rather limited, results in cancer therapy have been more impressive. He describes the major strategies that have been adopted up to date to make use of gene transfer for the therapy of malignant disease.

From the presentations of Smith and Brenner, it is clear that while admitting that many problems remain, they are both rather optimistic about the future of somatic gene therapy research. This rather optimistic view contrasts, however, to the more pessimistic one put forward recently (at a symposium in Los Angeles on March 20, 1998) by the well-known gene therapy researcher W. French Anderson: "The unfortunate fact is that, with the exception of a few anecdotal cases, there is no evidence of a gene therapy protocol that helps in any disease situation." However, he said this not in order to discourage further research. On the contrary, he takes this as an incentive to develop germ-line gene therapy.[6] As James Watson, codiscoverer of the double helix and the first Director of the US Human Genome Project, said at the same symposium, "[o]ne thing that seems pretty obvious is that germline therapy will probably be much more successful than somatic. If we wait for the success of somatic we'll wait until the sun burns out."[7]

History and its lessons

However, it is important with historical perspectives, not just forward-looking ones. In his paper, the philosopher LeRoy Walters looks both to the past and to the future: first,18 years back, then, 18 years ahead. Finally, he steps back to the early decades of this century and discusses the issue of eugenics. In his overview, he presents not only the scientific aspects but also ethical considerations and policy-making. Let me very briefly focus on some of Walters' historical remarks, leaving his futuristic part to the reader.

Why look back precisely18 years (starting 1998)? The reason is, of course, that in 1980 the first experiment on gene therapy was carried out by Martin Cline. This experiment was, however, premature and unauthorized, and it was one of the contributing factors which in1984 led to the attachment of a working group on gene therapy to the NIH Recombinant DNA Advisory Committee (RAC). A year later the RAC came forward with the first version of its "Points to consider", i.e. guidelines for somatic gene therapy. As chair of the working group, Walters was one of those who contributed to the articulation of these guidelines, and in his present paper he discusses its key ideas. The first gene therapy protocol was approved by the RAC in 1990.

In his final section, Walters turns to the eugenics in the US and Germany in the first half of this century. This issue is, of course, of special relevance to the issue of ethics and genetics. Many geneticists in the beginning of this century thought that social responsibility implied that they should support eugenic practices. Today most geneticists would say that social responsibility implies fighting eugenics. However, as Walters tries to show, the question is not quite as simple. The issue of preventing the transmission of genetic diseases to future generations might come to the forefront of the discussion once again, when we sometime in the future start to develop germ-line gene therapy. According to Walters, this is a good thing. He has (with Palmer) elsewhere defended germ-line gene therapy as a kind of voluntary "public-health program."[8]

In his paper, the historian of science Charles Weiner puts human gene therapy into another historical perspective by analyzing the debate on genetic engineering in the1960s and 70s. He finds that while a few scientists, such as Arne Tiselius and Jonathan Beckwith, took the social and ethical implications of this new technology seriously, many other scientists did not. Many scientists did not want a public debate out of fear for an "overreaction" that would interfere with their research and its funding. Many narrowed their ethical concerns to the immediate technical problems of laboratory safety and developed technical solutions to these problems, largely ignoring the ethical issues related to the possible applications of the findings. They separated the technical from the ethical. They focused on the means rather than the ends. Moreover, Weiner stresses that the commercialization of academic biology in the 1980s has created conflicts of interest that may seriously erode public trust. According to Weiner, all this have implications for present-day genetic research such as the Human Genome Project and gene therapy research.

Weiner concludes his paper by proposing certain guidelines for consideration in public decision-making regarding human genetic intervention. These include: disclosure of potential conflicts of interest, avoidance of genetic determinism and reductionism, prioritizing public health needs rather than commercial profit, and development of public literacy and a stronger sense of social responsibility among scientists.

Conceptual issues

Gene therapy raises certain conceptual questions. In her contribution, Sigrid Graumann, biologist and ethicist, criticizes certain basic conceptual presumptions of somatic gene therapy research. These presumptions are called "the central genetic dogma" by Francis Crick, codiscoverer of the double helix. The presumptions are that the phenotype is the realization of the genotypic program, that the base sequence is a simple code, and that the only direction of information is from DNA via RNA to protein. Graumann interprets this central genetic dogma as part of the leading paradigm, in a Kuhnian sense, of genetic research, and argues that this paradigm is now in a Kuhnian stage of crisis. She questions all the presumptions and argues that the effects of somatic gene transfer cannot be predicted with certainty. This holds for positive effects as well as negative ones. Therefore, somatic gene therapy can never be particularly successful and clinically useful. And this has, of course, ethical implications. Is it morally responsible to carry out gene transfer when the results cannot be predicted with a reasonable degree of certainty?

It seems possible to apply Graumann's argument to the above mentioned rather pessimistic view of some leading scientists regarding somatic gene therapy. Viewed from this perspective, Graumann's criticism implies that the limited success depends on the invalidity of certain basic presumptions.

The feminist theologian Karen Lebacqz discusses an even more fundamental conceptual issue, namely the concept of "therapy". She argues that this concept is irrevocably ambiguous. What counts as "therapy" to the dominant group in society may be an undesired intervention to marginalized groups such as blind people, deaf people, or people of very short stature. Disability is a social construct. What is considered a "disability" from the dominant culture is not necessarily a disability to those who deviate from the cultural norm. Moreover, Lebacqz stresses that even where intervention is accepted it might be ambiguous. The "self" that emerges following therapy may not be altogether comfortable. The sense of personal identity may have a tendency to remain with the untreated self. According to Lebacqz, the conclusion is that instead of "gene therapy" we should talk about "genetic intervention".

The ambiguity of "therapy" has also feminist implications. Therapy presupposes a conceptual distinction between normal and abnormal. Women have always deviated from the "normal" in the male-dominated society. Lebacqz argues that there is a risk that in a gene-focused society the normality of men and abnormality of women is seen as based in the genes. Society becomes "geneticized". The norms are being established with reference to genetics. This constitutes are more basic danger than the discrimination of women itself.

The ethicist Eric Juengst analyses the conceptual distinction between treatment and enhancement. Traditionally, this distinction has served as a major policy boundary where treatment is viewed as acceptable and enhancement as unacceptable. However, the distinction is not clear. Juengst finds at least three different ways of explicating it: professional domain accounts, normalcy accounts, and disease-based accounts. None of them is able to sustain a clear distinction between treatment and enhancement. However, no matter how the line is drawn, there is always a risk of "off-label" uses, i.e. uses other than the therapeutic applications originally intended in research. Therefore, the really important policy problem, according to Juengst, becomes how to control the access and use of gene transfer technologies, not how to control their research and development. How can the government see to it that social injustice and discrimination are avoided?

National perspectives: Germany and Japan

In the discussion of genetics and gene therapy it is important to recognize the cultural context. It is important to be aware of similarities and differences between different countries in attitudes, policies and so forth. In this book, the contributors come from many different countries: USA, Germany, Belgium, Japan, and Sweden. At the conference, even more nations were represented, including Russia.

One section of this volume is devoted to the national perspectives of Germany and Japan. These two countries are particularly interesting from a historical point of view, because of their eugenics policies in the past. In Germany, the Nazi eugenics still affects the discussion on genetics. People associate genetics with eugenics. In Japan, where a eugenic law was in force until just recently, social stigma linked to certain genetic diseases still remain. An understanding of the cultural context is particularly essential in order to understand the debate on gene therapy in these two countries.

In his paper, the theologian Dietmar Mieth presents some viewpoints and arguments which are typical for the German debate on gene therapy. The special character of the debate depends on certain factors that are peculiar to Germany. These factors include: the specific history of the country which requires sensitivity to phenomena like "selection", the legal prohibition against experimentation on human embryos, the impact of ecology on religious movements etc. Mieth stresses that the German debate has focused almost completely on germ-line gene therapy. In general, the view has been very restrictive.

The lawyer Rihito Kimura represents a Japanese perspective. In his paper, he describes the typical Japanese attitude of dependency to superiors, professionals and parents, which radically contrasts to the attitude of self-determination in Western culture. This mentality affects health care as well. It tends to prevent straightforward communication regarding disease between patients and physicians. This has, of course, implications for the clinical use of genetic diagnosis and gene therapy. However, traditional values are rapidly changing to more individualistic decision-making, and Kimura presents the Japanese Gene Therapy Guidelines from 1994 which stress the importance of informed consent.

Testing, screening, selecting, treating, preventing

The papers in the final section relate gene therapy to different kinds of genetic testing. The first paper asks about the influence of gene therapy on genetic screening. The second one discusses different types of gene therapy and suggests towards the end preimplantation genetic diagnosis (PGD) followed by embryo selection as an alternative to germ-line gene therapy. The third paper gives an extensive comparison between gene therapy and preselection based on PGD.

The ethicist Kris Dierickx anticipates that gene therapy might have far-reaching consequences for genetic screening. Genetic screening may be considered an obstacle for the development of gene therapy, because selective abortion on the basis of such screening might be a less expensive alternative. Moreover, gene therapy may sharpen the requirements for genetic screening. Once gene therapy becomes available, requirements such as reliable test methods, informed consent, and respect for privacy and confidentiality, will be considered more important. Finally, for some diseases, gene therapy may be considered the only missing factor in order to implement a genetic screening programme.

In his discussion of different kinds of gene therapy, the ethicist Nikolaus Knoepffler takes as a starting point the Kantian notion of human dignity. On this ethical basis, he finds somatic gene therapy morally unproblematic but germ-line gene therapy unacceptable. With regard to germ-line gene therapy, he stresses that in most cases we can reach the goal of avoiding the birth of children with genetic disease in a simpler and already clinically established way by PGD and embryo selection.

In his paper, the philosopher Christian Munthe compares gene therapy and preselection of embryos based on PGD. Gene therapy means that someone gets medical treatment. In preselection, however, the potential patient is exchanged for another individual who is not in need of any treatment. Munthe discusses to what extent the arguments for and against these kinds of genetic intervention apply equally to both of them. May the same benefits be achieved? Are fears for eugenics more warranted for gene therapy than preselection? Moreover, Munthe finds that preselection is an intervention on the germ-line and that it is presently clinically applied. This prompts him to ask how it is possible to argue that clinical application of germ-line gene therapy should not be permitted.

Conclusion

As is clear already from this brief overview, the papers of the volume are quite diverse. Many different views and perspectives are presented. Hopefully, however, the bringing together of various scientific, historical, conceptual, national, as well as ethical aspects of gene therapy, may create a better basis for reaching a well-considered standpoint. But it is beyond the scope of this volume to present such a standpoint. It is an issue for further study and dialogue.

Acknowledgments

I would like to thank the other two members of the planning committee of the conference "Gene Therapy: Ethical, Legal, and Social Perspectives" Professor Ulf G. Pettersson and Associate Professor Mats G. Hansson. I would also like to thank Professor LeRoy Walters at The Kennedy Institute of Ethics in Washington DC for good collaboration, likewise The Department of Public Health and Caring Sciences at Uppsala University. Moreover, I am grateful to David Kronlid for practical assistance in organizing the conference and to Pernilla Parenmalm for practical help in editing this volume. Finally, I would like to thank the Board of the Centre for Research Ethics for taking the initiative to the conference in the first place. This holds in particular for the former Chair of the Board Professor Carl-Henric Grenholm.

Financial support of the conference has been provided by The Swedish Medical Research Council, The Swedish Council for Research in Humanities and Social Sciences, The Swedish Council for Planning and Coordination of Research, The ELSA Group in Sweden, The Swedish Cancer Society, and the Kennedy Institute of Ethics (Washington DC). The publication of the book has been funded by The ELSA Group.

Notes

1. Orkin, S. H., Motulsky, A. D., 1995. *Report and Recommendations of the Panel to Assess the NIH Investment in Research on Gene Therapy*. URL: www.nih.gov/od/oba; Stock, G., Campbell, J., 1998. *Summary Report: Engineering the Human Germline Symposium*. URL: www.ess.ucla.edu:80/huge/.
2. Walters, 1986.
3. For a recent overview of the main arguments, see Holtug, 1997.
4. Richter, Bachetta, 1998, pp. 304–306.
5. Orkin, Motulsky, 1995. URL: www.nih.gov/od/oba.
6. Stock, Campbell, 1998. URL: www.ess.ucla.edu:80/huge/.
7. Ibid.
8. Walters, Palmer, 1997, p. 88.

Bibliography

Holtug, N., 1997. "Altering Humans: The Case For and Against Human Gene Therapy." *Cambridge Quaterly of Health Care Ethics* 6, pp. 157–174.

Richter, G., Bachetta, M. D., 1998. "Interventions in the Human Genome: Some Moral and Ethical Considerations." *Journal of Medicine and Philosophy* 23, 3, pp. 303–317.

Walters, L., 1986. "The Ethics of Human Gene Therapy." *Nature* 320, pp. 225–227.

Walters, L., Palmer, J. G., 1997. *The Ethics of Human Gene Therapy.* Oxford University Press: Oxford.

Science

C. I. EDVARD SMITH

Gene Therapy: A Molecular Perspective

What is the genetic material and how does it function?

Gene therapy is a form of applied molecular biology. The vast knowledge on genetic material that has been gathered over the past fifty years has gradually paved the way for developing technologies of gene transfer into humans. The genetic material consists in the main of DNA which is copied into RNA, which subsequently serves as a blue-print for the making of proteins. In humans the DNA is formed by 3 billion ($10^{9)}$ base pairs forming the haploid genome, whereas viruses may contain only a few thousand of these building blocks. Certain organisms instead use RNA as their primary source of genetic information. Some proteins have mainly a structural function, such as forming the cytoskeleton in the cell, whereas others display signalling or enzymatic activities. In many proteins several functions are integrated. Thus, in a genetic disease the primary abnormality is to be found in the DNA, whereas the actual disease phenotype is caused by protein abnormalities that occur secondarily.

Which diseases are potential targets for gene therapy?

In human genetic diseases, a protein may be lacking as a consequence of a mutation in the corresponding gene (DNA). An example of such a disease is cystic fibrosis, in which mutations in a cell membrane ion channel gene, predisposes for bacterial infections which cause lung damage. In tumors genetic changes occur, which may sometimes be inherited, but are most often acquired. Typically, mutations in several different genes are needed for tumor development. Moreover, infectious diseases, such as the one caused by the human immunodeficiency virus (HIV), are due to the transfer of viral genetic material into the patient cells (in this case viral RNA is converted into DNA in the patient cell). However, gene therapy is not limited to genetic disease. The transfer of genes could be envisaged also for non-genetic disease, simply as a way to deliver a drug. In this case the properties of DNA makes it a drug through its capacity to serve as a template for protein synthesis.

How does gene therapy work?

In a patient with a defective gene, the ideal situation would be if it was possible to repair this gene. However, with the present technology this is not feasible. Instead a functional, extra copy of the gene is normally added. In patients with a dominantly inherited disease, a functional copy of the gene already exists. Here, the addition of a second normal copy may not be sufficient to change the disease phenotype. Thus with current gene therapy methods, dominantly inherited diseases are not considered to be good targets. In some diseases it may be necessary to target essentially every single cell with a mutation, whereas in other diseases a cell carrying a functional copy of the corresponding gene may display a survival advantage as compared to cells only having defective genes. Here it may suffice to correct very few cells and still obtain functional correction.

Which are the desired properties of a system transferring genetic material?

In the same way as different diseases display divergent phenotypes, the type of gene therapy differs considerably depending on the target disease. In some cases the aim is to maintain a stable function of the transferred genetic material; in other cases, a continued template function would instead be detrimental. In these latter cases a transient function is needed. For a stable function, the integration of the transferred genetic material to the endogenous DNA has been considered the optimal solution. Human DNA is located in the chromosomes within the cell nucleus. To obtain a persistent function, methods have been developed to transfer genes into chromosomes. Conversely, for transient function, DNA vehicles, also called vectors, that will only be active during days or weeks have been developed. These vectors do not integrate into chromosomes, but instead exist as separate molecules, called episomes.

A challenge in the gene therapy field has been to develop efficient gene transfer systems. It should be possible to produce large amounts of the genetic material to be transferred, and also to efficiently package the DNA into relevant vectors. Once the DNA has entered the cell it should exert its function during the desired time. The existing vector systems are suboptimal as the degree of gene transfer is often poor. Even if an adequate amount of DNA is transferred it frequently will only function for a limited time period. Another desired feature of vectors is a targeting function. Thus, ideally one would like to inject the vector, e.g. into the blood stream, after which the vector would bind to its target tissue and thereby selectively deliver the gene to the relevant tissue.

Which transfer techniques are available today?

The method of choice for transferring DNA to human cells is to employ derivatives of viruses. The general principle is to isolate a virus with appropriate properties, remove viral genetic elements that can cause harm, insert the therapeutic gene and let the virus use its natural way of infecting the human cells. Certain viruses will integrate their genetic material into chromosomes, whereas others will not. Some viruses will only be able to harbour relatively short DNA sequences, thereby disqualifying certain genes from transfer. Other viruses may induce immune responses in the infected individual obviating efficient transfer.

It is also possible to simply transfer the DNA itself in the absence of any viral proteins. Here size is no limitation allowing the transfer of any gene. However, viruses have developed a very efficient transport system for genetic material. In comparison, the transfer of naked DNA is very inefficient. It is likely that in the future mixtures of synthetic viral proteins and genetic material will be used. These mixtures would have properties more resembling what we normally relate to as drugs.

Ethical considerations

The ethical considerations may naturally address many different aspects. From a more gene transfer technological point of view, the following points may be identified: Somatic cells versus germ cells, risks for the patient, risks for non-patients, and what distinguishes a disease from a character?

If a gene is inserted into a germ cell (egg cell or sperm) it will for ever stay in the genome of this individual and be transferred to the children. From a strictly technical point of view, current technologies do not allow repair, but instead the transferred gene could end up anywhere in the genome. This is what happens in transgenic animals. Here the gene frequently behaves as expected, but may be silenced and could potentially display undesired properties. Moreover, once a gene has been inserted into germ cells it cannot be removed. In contrast, when a gene is inserted into somatic cells it cannot be transferred to the off-spring, but will only remain as long as the recipient stays alive. In families in which a genetic disease exists, in vitro-fertilization, combined with the selection of healthy fertilized eggs is frequently technically feasible. There are some families where this is not possible due to that there are no healthy genes to select from. However, from a practical point of view these families are very rare exceptions, constituting only a very minor proportion.

When a gene is inserted into the genome of any cell it may function abnormally, or could affect adjacent genes causing them to misbehave. Although insertion mutagenesis causing tumor formation has so far not been seen in humans there is a potential risk. As discussed the viral vectors are normally created by removing harmful sequences and replacing them with the therapeutic gene. The more alterations that have been made, the less is the chance that recombinations could revert the virus into a wild-type form. However, the risk is never completely eliminated. This also means that there could be a potential risk for non-patients. However, for all practical purposes this risk has been considered essentially non-existing for the current generation of vectors.

At present gene therapy is only considered for severe diseases. In the future it is likely that gene therapy will develop into a much more efficient tool with few side effects. At this point in time the indications for gene therapy are likely to be widened. Although there is often a general consensus for the use of the word "disease" when discussing severe forms of illness, it is obvious that when less severe forms could become potential targets, one may eventually reach a level where there is a no longer a general agreement on whether a phenomenon should be classified as a disease or as a character.

MALCOLM BRENNER

Gene Therapy: At Present and in the Future

Applications of gene therapy

At first, it was assumed that gene therapy would be used to correct traditional single gene disorders. The original target diseases included inherited immune deficiencies, hemoglobinopathies (such as sickle cell disease), and cystic fibrosis. If this was indeed the only application of gene transfer, there would be few moral or ethical dilemmas in adopting the procedure. Moreover, since such conditions form less than 2% of human disease, the overall impact of gene transfer on public health would have been limited. However, it quickly became apparent that defective genes could be replaced not only in inherited single gene defects, but also in diseases in which a multiplicity of genes contribute to disease predisposition or in which the genetic disorder is acquired. One example of the latter application is cancer, which is caused by several genetic abnormalities within the malignant cell. But potentially the greatest importance of gene transfer lies in its ability to modify the function of a cell, providing it with an ability that it previously never possessed, or removing a function of which the cell would normally be capable. When one considers these additional possibilities, it quickly becomes apparent that gene transfer may have an impact on almost every disease. Hence, there is increasing interest in using gene transfer not only for the treatment of inherited and acquired genetic disorders, but also to treat degenerative conditions and infectious diseases. Overall, it is difficult to conceive of any disease in which gene transfer might not be able to play a substantive role.

The applications of gene therapy go beyond the treatment of disease. It is axiomatic that disease *prevention* produces more cost effective and patient effective result than disease *treatment*. As the Human Genome Project and associated studies begin to reveal genetic predispositions to a wide range of common disorders, the desire to use gene transfer as "geno-prevention" will steadily increase. Moreover, as we understand more and more about human cellular biology and the ways in which different patterns of cell growth and differentiation can modify the overall function of the individual, the temptation to use gene transfer to produce "enhanced" human beings will become ever greater. It is in these areas of enhancement that ethical and moral concerns are particularly substantive.

An additional area of concern is germ-line gene therapy. To date, all gene therapy practiced has been somatic gene therapy. That is, the cells of the existing individual are altered, but there is no transfer of the altered genetic material to germ cells or to any offspring. In other words, the gene dies with the modified individual. The concept of germ line gene therapy, in which altered function is handed down through successive generations, is much more problematic, both scientifically and ethically, and will be dealt with briefly towards the end of this chapter.

Gene therapy for non-malignant diseases

Although the potential for gene therapy is therefore enormous—and has been accompanied by equally massive hyperbole—the reality is that current gene therapy technologies are extraordinarily primitive and ineffective. For the types of applications outlined above, it will be necessary to devise greatly improved vectors (gene transfer agents). They will need to be targeted to the desired cell, not only in terms of reaching the cell surface, but also in their ability to enter the cell nucleus. If vectors are to integrate in the host cell DNA, it is also desirable that they should be targeted to specific safe areas within the genome so that they do not disrupt normal cellular functions. In addition, gene transfer should be highly efficient so that the majority of targeted cells are corrected or modified. Gene transfer should also be safe and (for most applications) the product of the new gene should be controlled in terms of quantity, timing and site. Although there are many viral and non-viral vectors currently available, none of them even begin to attain many of these desirable characteristics. While the vectors used to date have been reasonably safe in the great majority of patients, they have been entirely untargeted and inefficient, and regulation of the transgene is only now beginning to become feasible. These inadequacies have severely constrained the clinical applications of gene transfer. In non-malignant disease, investigators have focused on conditions in which correction of a small number of cells may be of benefit, either because the corrected cells have a growth advantage over the uncorrected cells and may therefore repopulate the individual, or because even small quantities of the transgene product are beneficial. It has also been critical to chose diseases in which unregulated expression would be safe and effective. Hence, the first disease chosen to be treated by gene transfer was adenosine deaminase deficiency, a form of severe combined immunodeficiency. In this condition, ADA corrected cells have a growth advantage over uncorrected cells, there is no requirement for gene regulation, and relatively small amounts of gene product can be beneficial. Patients with ADA deficiency have been treated in two ways; either by the administration of T lymphocytes containing the transgene, or by infusion of gene modified cord blood progenitor cells which are anticipated to differentiate into ADA containing T cells. Although several patients appear to have sustained some immunologic benefit from this approach, as yet there is no definitive evidence that the treatment has been curative. In particular, in patients receiving the transduced cord blood cells, only limited numbers of gene corrected lymphocytes circulated, and immune function was incompletely restored. Limited benefits have been obtained in other inherited conditions such as Fanconi anemia (complementation group C) and Gaucher's disease. In all, gene transfer has been attained but at levels too low for unequivocal benefit. Other diseases, such as cystic fibrosis, have proved even more refractory, with only the most modest evidence of gene transfer and no evidence at all for clinical benefit. Such poor results are understandable, since in most diseases there is no selective advantage for the minority population of transduced cells over their untransduced neighbors. Recently, more hopeful preclinical data have been generated that suggest that injection of virus vectors into muscle can produce sufficient quantities of Factor IX to treat patients with deficiencies of this clotting component, and clinical trials of the approach are ongoing. Studies using gene transfer vectors encoding vascular growth factors have also produced promising results in patients with peripheral vascular disease. These are now being investigated in patients with coronary artery disease, where they have also been reported to provide benefit. Given the limited activity of current vectors, this last approach, which requires only localized and transient production of small quantities of the gene product, may have a higher chance of success than the more ambitious alternatives first tried.

Gene therapy for malignant diseases

While the benefits of gene therapy for non-malignant conditions have generally been rather limited, results in cancer therapy have (somewhat surprisingly) been more impressive. To date, four major strategies have been adopted to make use of gene transfer for the therapy of malignant disease.

1) Modifying the tumor itself by:
   i) repairing one or more of the genetic defects associated with the malignant process
   ii) delivering a pro-drug metabolizing enzyme that will render the tumor sensitive to the corresponding cytotoxic pro-drug agent
   iii) introducing a gene that will trigger an anti-tumor immune response.

2) Modifying the immune response to the tumor by altering the specificity or effector function of immune systems cells.
3) Decreasing the sensitivity of normal host tissue, by delivering genes that render the tissue resistant to cytotoxic drugs and thereby increase the therapeutic index of cytotoxic agents.
4) Marking normal and malignant hematopoietic cells to track them in vivo and thereby more closely monitor the efficacy of more conventional therapies. Some examples of each approach follow.

The first major strategy is modification of the tumor. There is an attractive elegance to the strategy of introducing genetic material into a malignancy to correct the specific genetic defects that contribute to the malignant phenotype. A number of mutant oncogenes and fusion genes have been described in malignant disease that are certainly specific to the abnormal clone, and the products of which may be a critical component of the malignant process. Unfortunately, this approach is technologically extremely demanding. All malignancies are the result of a multiplicity of genetic abnormalities, so that correction of a single one would need to be a lethal event for the cell in order for benefit to be obtained. Moreover, many relevant gene defects produce molecules with "transdominant effects" that will continue to produce a malignant phenotype even if the wild-type gene is introduced. Such transdominant genes can only be neutralized by introducing antisense RNA, by ribozymes or by homologous recombination with a wild-type gene. None of these approaches are fully evolved. Finally, present methods of gene transfer are inefficient and are unlikely to be sufficient to produce lasting benefits. Notwithstanding the above limitations, several protocols are under way using a tumor correction approach. In spite of the polygenic etiology of cancer, it is hoped that certain individual genetic abnormalities will be both pivotal to the malignant process and amenable to correction. Perhaps the most widely used molecule for this approach is a wild-type p53 gene. This was initially used to correct lung cancers with an abnormal p53, but has subsequently been applied to tumors in which p53 is entirely normal. Unexpectedly, given the low level of gene transfer, significant tumor responses have been seen when these genes have been delivered by adenoviruses to lung cancers and to head and neck tumors. It may be that a small number of dying transduced cells can trigger an immunologic or other bystander effect that would result in much more widespread destruction. Interest is also increasing in targeting the genetic pathways involved in regulating apoptosis, since experimental models suggest that even minor perturbations in these pathways can greatly modify the sensitivity of cancer cells to chemotherapy and radiotherapy. Hence, it may be possible to use combinations of gene therapy with conventional therapy to produce an enhanced response.

Instead of introducing genes that modify genetic defects in tumors, efforts have been made to insert genes that will encode enzymes able to convert harmless prodrugs into lethal cytotoxins. The first clinical studies introduced a thymidine kinase (Tk) gene into tumor cells using a retroviral vector. On exposure to ganciclovir, the transduced cells will phosphorlate the drugs. If the cell then divides, the active compound will be incorporated into DNA with lethal consequences. Subsequently this approach has been extended using adenoviruses to deliver the Tk gene, and has now been used for a wide range of tumors, including those of brain, prostate and ovary. Some tumor responses have been reported and, once again, the degree of response seems greatly to exceed the level of gene transfer. For Tk, there is a well established bystander effect which is produced both by the transfer of toxic molecules through gap junctions between modified and unmodified cells and also by an immunological mechanism developing in response to antigens released by the small proportion of cells that are directly killed by the gene product. A number of other prodrug systems, including cytosine deaminase, have been described and these are now entering clinical trials.

Because of the limited efficacy of gene transfer and the inability to target vectors directly to cancer cells, efforts have been made to recruit the immune system to compensate for these deficiencies. It is now apparent that tumors may contain a number of unique or tumor-associated antigens and that these antigens may be processed into peptides within the cell and expressed on the cell surface in combination with HLA molecules. In this form they can be recognized by T lymphocytes. If a tumor cell is a relatively weak immunogen, then gene transfer may serve to enhance the immunogenicity of the tumor associated antigens it expresses. An immune response so generated may then be able to recognize and destroy non-transduced tumor cells expressing the same tumor associated antigens elsewhere in the body. A range of immunstimulatory molecules have been studied, including cytokine genes such as IL2 and GM-CSF, allogeneic MHC molecules and costimulatory molecules such as B7.1 and CD40 Ligand. Certainly in animal models these approaches all produce the desired immunostimulation, and more than one hundred clinical studies are now underway in a range of different malignancies. The results to date can be summarized as showing a significant increase in immune reactivity to the tumors with occasional substantial anti-tumor responses, including complete remissions. As efforts are made to enhance the functionality of this approach by combining different classes of immunogenic molecules, it is hoped that a higher proportion of responders will be observed. In addition, once patients have made responses it is possible to isolate tumor specific antibody and T cell receptor molecules from these individuals. These reagents can then be utilized in secondary studies where they can be given directly to patients and further therapeutic benefit obtained.

Now, we come to the second major strategy: modification of the host immune system. As alluded to above, it is possible to obtain genetically modified T lymphocytes that recognize tumor cells. One of the simplest examples of this is to eradicate EBV-associated malignancies such as immunoblastic and Hodgkin lymphomas using genetically marked T lymphocytes that are specific for Epstein-Barr virus. Because of the presence of a genetic marker, these anti-tumor T cells can be tracked in vivo and shown to persist long term, to infiltrate EBV positive tumors and to destroy the EBV infected malignant cells. Extensions of this approach, using T cells transduced to express other tumor specific receptors are now in progress, for example in patients with colon cancer.

The third strategy is modification of host cytotoxic drug sensitivity. Our increased understanding of the mechanisms of cytotoxic drug action, and the methods of resistance to this action have suggested gene therapy approaches to protect normal host tissues from the toxicity of chemotherapy. It is hoped that the increased or prolonged administration of cytotoxic drugs that would then be possible would be able to cure a higher proportion of patients. The MDR1 gene has been the most widely considered for human therapy. The product of this gene, P-glycoprotein, functions as a drug efflux pump and can produce resistance to many chemotherapeutic agents. Gene transfer of the MDR1 gene in murine hematopoietic stem cells permits them to expand and repopulate the mouse following administration of otherwise lethal doses of cytotoxic drugs. Although human studies have begun with this gene, the results to date have been disappointing, with limited evidence for enhanced survival of the transduced cells on administration of the selective cytotoxic agent. For a variety of reasons, however, MDR1 may not be the optimal gene to use, and there is hope that alternative drug resistance molecules, such as dihydrofolate reductase mutants, will be more satisfactory.

Finally, gene marking has also been valuable, not in the direct therapy of cancer, but in tracking the response of patients to therapy and in discovering why these responses failed. Some examples include the use of gene marking to detect the source of relapse after autologous bone marrow transplantation and to track the survival and efficacy of infused anti-tumor specific T cells (see above). It is likely that marking studies will continue to be used as a means of monitoring cellular therapies such as bone marrow transplantation and cytotoxic T lymphocytes.

Germ-line gene therapy and genetic enhancement

The applications of somatic gene therapy described to date have been relatively non-controversial. Ethical problems will begin to arise when gene transfer is used to produce "cosmetic" changes including mental or physical enhancement, and will become greater still when it is feasible to move from somatic to germ-line gene therapy. While it might be tempting to simply place a complete and permanent ban on any germ-line gene therapy, this would be inappropriate. There are genetic diseases for which correction in postembryonic life is simply too late; the associated developmental abnormalities have devastating or even lethal consequences that cannot be corrected even by the presence of a normally functioning gene. In other diseases, the ability to correct target cells located over a wide anatomical distribution may not be feasible once the embryo reaches a certain size and complexity. This last consideration would also be important when gene transfer is used for the correction of any genetic predisposition to disorders that may occur in several different organ systems. For example, patients with BRCA1 are predisposed to tumors of the breast and the ovary. In these cases, the simplest way of disease prevention is to correct an embryo as soon as possible after fertilization! At present, there is little pressure from patients or investigators to perform germ line gene therapy, because of a lack of technical capabilities. There is a need to develop successful methods for homologous recombination (insertion of the gene of interest to directly replace the gene that is considered abnormal or suboptimal) and to develop techniques to perform QA/QC on the apparently corrected embryo. Once these techniques are in place, however, there will be a strong impetus to correct genes that adversely affect development. The use of germ line gene therapy to prevent clearly defined diseases is probably justified, and in many countries there will be only limited societal concerns for this application. However, difficulties will arise for conditions, ranging from short stature to early baldness, that have a genetic basis, but are not genuine "diseases". As we begin to understand more and more about the developmental biology of humans, the desire to produce germ line enhancement of mental and physical functions will become ever greater, with many deeply troubling implications. While the ethical and moral issues of enhancement certainly need to be carefully considered, these "therapies" are not imminent. First of all, our knowledge of the genetics of developmental biology is inadequate to achieve substantial enhancement. Secondly, gene transfer technology is far below that which would be necessary for safe and effective enhancement. Finally, few of the characteristics which we would wish to enhance, from stature to intelligence, are likely to be the products of single genes. A multiplicity of germ line modifications would need to be made for any desired difference to occur in the resulting individual, a task that is far beyond current abilities. Nonetheless, these restraints are technological rather than conceptual. Eventually the problems will be solved and the potential will become reality. It is therefore important to have in place a set of ethical and moral guidelines for all involved in this field.

Bibliography

Brenner, M. K. 1996. "Gene transfer in haematological malignancy." *Ann. Med.* 28, p. 491.

Crystal, R. G., 1995. "Transfer of genes to humans: early lessons and obstacles to success." *Science* 270, p. 404.

Gordon, J. W., 1998. "Germline alteration by gene therapy: assessing and reducing the risks." *Mol. Med. Today* 4, p. 468.

Mulligan, R. C., 1993. "The basic science of gene therapy." *Science* 260, p. 926.

Sadelain, M., 1997. "Genetic treatment of the haemoglobinopathies: recombinations and new combinations." *Br. J. Haematol.* 98, p. 247.

Wivel, N. A., Wilson, J.M., 1998. "Methods of gene delivery." *Hematol. Oncol. Clin. North. Am.* 12, p. 483.

History and Its Lessons

LEROY WALTERS

Human Gene Therapy: Past, Present, and Future

My remarks will be divided into three parts. First, I will look back on the past 18 years, the period between 1980 and 1998, and to the early history of somatic cell gene therapy. Second, I will attempt to look toward the future—to the next 18 years—and to explore what might happen between now and the year 2016. Third, I would like to compare the issues surrounding current human gene therapy and future human genetic intervention with the issues that arose in the first half of the 20th century surrounding the eugenics movements in the United States and Germany.

Two cases

I will begin with patients and with two case studies. The first patient is David, "the boy in the bubble." He appeared on the cover of *People* magazine from October 29, 1984.[1] There was a continuation of this story in the next week's issue on November 5th. How many of you have heard of him?

David was born with an X-linked type of severe combined immune deficiency. That means that both parts of his immune system were disabled from the time of birth. David was born in September of 1971. He had a sister who was four years older than he, and his parents had lost an older brother at the age of seven months, who, like David, had had severe combined immune deficiency. His parents knew when they conceived David that they were taking the risk of having another child with the same disease.

Two minutes after his birth, David was moved into an incubator and a sterile environment. That is where he remained, in various kinds of isolated settings, for the first 12 years of his life. Diagnostic tests soon after his birth indicated that David did indeed have the same severe combined immune deficiency that had killed his older brother.

David flourished in his protected environment, insofar as anyone could. Here is what his parents set up for him at home in the living room. Notice the eight-by-ten playroom; attached to that is a transport bubble in which David was contained as he was moved back and forth between home and the hospital.

Like most young people, David enjoyed playing with the hose in the backyard. Here he is at the age of about five, in a space suit designed by NASA specifically for him. The next slide shows David kissing his mother through a plastic barrier. This was as close as David and his mother could get, at the boundary of the transport bubble.

In 1983, with the progress that had been made with bone marrow transplantation, David's family decided to try to liberate him from the bubble. His sister was the closest match, genetically and immunologically, and she agreed to provide bone marrow, which was harvested in Boston and flown to Houston. David received the bone marrow transplant late on October 21, 1983. Then the family waited and hoped.

The family celebrated Christmas at home together, and even though there was no evidence that the transplant had taken, they were still optimistic. On New Year's Day 1984, David began to run a slight fever, and his clinical course from then through mid-February went downhill very rapidly. On February 22nd, David was taken out of the bubble so that his physicians could treat him more intensively. He died later that day.[2]

It was about a year later that David's immunologist, William Shearer, and his colleagues published an article in the *New England Journal of Medicine*, looking back on David's case.[3] Dr. Shearer and his fellow clinicians had discovered at autopsy why David's clinical course had deteriorated so precipitously. Unbeknownst to anyone, the bone marrow from David's sister harbored a silent Epstein-Barr virus. Her normally functioning immune system kept the Epstein-Barr virus suppressed. In David's body, with no functioning immune system, the Epstein-Barr virus had no opposition and caused a fulminant B-cell lymphoma, which killed David within just a few months.

What makes this an incredibly sad case is that everyone involved did everything they could do at the time: the family (and especially the older sister), who made all the accommodations they could; the best physicians in the world, who were taking care of him; and David himself, who exhibited enormous courage. There is a sense in which David was born about ten years too soon.

The major artifact that remains from David's life is the plastic transport bubble shown in the next slide. This bubble is not currently on display, but it is owned by the National Museum of American History at the Smithsonian Institution, in Washington, D.C. On the slide you can see some of David's books and the size and shape of the transport bubble. Here is another view of the transport bubble with the little commode, canned foods, water, children's books.

The second case contrasts with David's, not solely because of gene therapy, I should acknowledge right away. The young woman on the right in this slide is named Ashanti DeSilva. She was born in 1986 with an autosomal recessive form of the same disease, severe combined immune deficiency. Her symptoms

	Somatic	Germ-Line
Cure or Prevention of Disease	1	2
Enhancement of Capabilities	3	4

Figure 1. *Four Types of Potential Genetic Intervention.*

and illnesses in her early years paralleled those of a patient with end-stage AIDS; it seemed as if every microbe in the environment attacked Ashanti's defenseless body and made her sick.

Both Ashanti and Cynthia Cutshall first received a synthetic enzyme called PEG-ADA, which helped. But in Ashanti DeSilva's case, in particular, the benefit from that enzyme gradually decreased. And in 1990, Ashanti DeSilva became the first patient to receive gene therapy in an approved protocol.

She appeared on a picture in *Time* magazine from June 7, 1993. There was an accompanying story by Larry Thompson entitled "The First Kids with New Genes" in the same issue.[4] Ashanti DeSilva was almost seven in the picture. I have since met her—in fact, we were on consecutive panels testifying at a congressional hearing. I think she must have been about nine at the time, and she was acting like a typical nine-year-old. She told her father she was very bored by the hearing and hoped they could get out of the hearing room just as soon as possible.

From all reports, both Ashanti DeSilva and Cynthia Cutshall currently enjoy lives that are as normal as the lives of any other adolescents.

Above is a two-by-two matrix that divides human genetic intervention into four possible subtypes (see Figure 1).

Across the top, you see the distinction between somatic interventions and germ-line interventions. Somatic interventions stop with the patient; they die with the patient, just as an organ that is transplanted into a patient would die with the patient. Along the side you see the distinction between the cure or prevention of disease, on the one hand, and the enhancement of capabilities. The vertical line is rather sharp and clear; a genetic change either affects only one generation, or it affects multiple generations and is passed down through a family line.

Later on, I will try to convince you that the horizontal line is not quite so sharp and clear and that certain activities can be described *either* as cure or prevention of disease *or* as enhancement, depending on how you look at them.

The past 18 years

Let us look back to the first 18 years of somatic cell human gene therapy. This will be a trip down memory lane for those of you familiar with the field. In 1980, President Carter received a letter from three religious leaders of Jewish, Catholic and Protestant religious communities.[5] This letter was sent shortly after the Supreme Court decision in *Diamond v. Chakrabarty*, which allowed the patenting of microorganisms, but the religious leaders also expressed concern about human genetic engineering and a "brave new world" just around the corner.

Later that year the *Los Angeles Times* reported that Dr. Martin Cline had tried gene therapy on two patients—one in Israel and one in Italy—without the permission of the IRB at UCLA.[6] Dr. Cline was punished following an investigation by the NIH. Soon after the story of Dr. Cline's experiment broke, W. French Anderson and John Fletcher published an article entitled "Human Gene Therapy: When Is It Ethical to Begin?" in *the New England Journal of Medicine*.[7] French Anderson told me in a later conversation that one reason he wanted to rush this article into print was to protect the field of gene therapy from an overreaction to Dr. Cline's premature experiment.

Was Dr. Cline's unapproved experiment premature? It definitely was premature. Dr. Cline was trying to treat a hemoglobin disorder, beta-zero thalassemia. Today, eighteen years after Dr. Cline treated his two patients, there still is not a gene therapy proposal going through the review process that aims to treat these kinds of disorders. They are much too complex for the early stages of human gene therapy.

In 1982, both Europe and the United States became concerned about genetic engineering. In January the Parliamentary Assembly of the Council of Europe adopted Receommendation 934 (1982) on genetic engineering.[8] Later in 1982 a U.S. presidential commission on bioethics produced a report entitled *Splicing Life*.[9] Less than two years later, in 1984, a working group on human gene therapy was attached to the NIH Recombinant DNA Advisory Committee, affectionately known as the RAC. In that same year, the Office of Technology Assessment, a congressional body, also produced a report titled *Human Gene Therapy: Background Paper*.[10] (Congress at that time had a way to look at the technologies of the future. For reasons that escape me, Congress, in the early 1990s, abolished the Office of Technology Assessment and therewith its ability to look ahead.)

In 1985, the first version of the Points to Consider document—really, guidelines for somatic cell gene therapy—was produced.[11] Those of us who were involved in that process were concerned to get this document finished because we thought the first gene therapy protocol might be just around the corner.

In 1986, the Institute of Medicine sponsored a meeting on human somatic cell gene therapy. Eve Nichols, now at the Whitehead Institute at MIT, was deeply involved in planning for the 1986 meeting. Ms. Nichols was the author of the 1988 book entitled *Human Gene Therapy*,[12] which has stood the test of time very well.

In that same year, the first gene-marking study was approved by the Human Gene Therapy Subcommittee (as it was by then called), and by the NIH RAC. In 1990, the first gene therapy studies were approved by the RAC. One of the protocols was for severe combined immune deficiency and was started in September of 1990; the other was for the treatment of cancer and was initiated in January 1991.

In 1992, the Human Gene Therapy Subcommittee was merged into the parent committee. There really was virtually nothing other than gene therapy for the RAC to consider; there were no more known biohazards of recombinant DNA research about which to worry. In some ways the early 1990s were the golden era for the review of gene therapy in a public policy forum.[13]

In 1994, matters began to become more complicated, in part because activists in the AIDS community complained that RAC review was requiring too much time, given the urgency of the worldwide epidemic, and in part because some pharmaceutical companies chafed under the discipline of the public review process. There was the risk of being embarrassed in a public question and answer session.

In autumn 1995, a committee under Inder Verma reported to NIH Director Harold Varmus and recommended that the RAC be continued but that it review only those protocols that raised novel issues.[14] That same fall, there was a sobering report by the Orkin-Motulsky panel on the NIH investment in gene therapy research.[15] This second report concluded that there had been almost no success to date in the field of gene therapy and that there was a real need to go back to the drawing board and do a great deal more basic biological research before attempting to treat patients.

In May, June, and early July of 1996, Dr. Varmus proposed to abolish the RAC. In July, several members of Congress, numerous academics, and some citizens protested this plan. In response, Dr. Varmus reversed his decision, retaining the RAC with somewhat modified functions. One year later, the RAC stopped approving and disapproving specific gene therapy protocols; that role is now with the Food and Drug Administration. In the fall of 1997, the RAC participated in planning the first gene therapy policy conference, to look at broader issues surrounding human genetics. The conference focused on genetic enhancement.

In February of 1998, the number of gene therapy protocols submitted to the NIH and the FDA reached 200—in addition to 30 gene-marking protocols and two non-therapeutic protocols in which vectors are being tried on normal volunteers.[16]

MEMBERS
WORKING GROUP ON HUMAN GENE THERAPY
NIH RECOMBINANT DNA ADVISORY COMMITTEE
January 1985

W. French Anderson — medicine
Judith Areen — law
Alexander M. Capron — law
James F. Childress — ethics
Samuel Gorovitz — ethics
Susan K. Gottesman — laboratory research
Maurice J. Mahoney — medicine
Robert E. Mitchell (RAC chair, ex officio) — law
Arno G. Motulsky — medicine
Robert F. Murray — medicine
Robert F. Rich — public policy
Harold Varmus — laboratory research
LeRoy Walters — ethics (working group chair)
Anne R. Witherby — layperson
William J. Gartland — executive secretary
Howard M. Temin, consultant — laboratory research

Figure 2.

Permit me to go back to 1984 and 1985, and to pay tribute to the people who worked so hard to develop guidelines for the gene therapy field. It was a decisively interdisciplinary group (see Figure 2). The Working Group included French Anderson in medicine; Alexander Capron in law; James Childress in ethics; Arno Motulsky in medicine; Harold Varmus (at the time, a laboratory researcher); and Anne Witherby, a layperson. The late Howard Temin, a Nobel laureate, served as a consultant to the group.

Out of the work of that group came a ten-page document called the 'Points to Consider.'[17] The 'Points' were not regulations; they were not even guidelines. They were, instead, approximately 110 questions that we asked investigators to answer as they thought about performing gene therapy in human patients. I will not attempt to cover all 110 questions but instead will reduce them to seven questions that I think capture the essence of what the Points to Consider document was trying to do.

Question 1: What is the disease to be treated, and what do we know about the natural history of the disease? Is it serious enough to merit this new kind of intervention?

Question 2: What alternative therapies are available? If there are reaonably effective existing therapies, as for phenylketonuria, then perhaps the disease is not a good early candidate for gene therapy. With severe combined immune deficiency there was considerable debate on the following question: Is the synthetic enzyme PEG-ADA so effective that we do not need to resort to gene therapy?

Question 3: What are the potential harms that could be caused by the gene therapy procedure? Here we as a Subcommittee asked the researchers for data from well-designed, well-controlled laboratory studies in animals or tissue culture.

Question 4: What are the potential benefits of the gene therapy procedure for the recipients? Here again, we asked not for pious hopes but for data about in vitro studies or laboratory animal studies that gave us a basis for concluding that there was at least a reasonable possibility of benefit to patients—or of gaining important information about potential toxicity.

These first four questions were all data-driven. There followed three other questions that were less dependent on data.

Question 5: What procedures will be followed to ensure fairness in the selection of recipients? For a rare disorder such as severe combined immune deficiency, that wasn't so difficult: patients were difficult to find, and almost every patient's family wanted to participate in a study. But when we received our first protocols for brain tumors, there was a rush of patients and families to get into the protocols, to be put into one of the first 10 or 20 slots in those studies. And there were occasions when state governors called the NIH Director's office or when the husband of a patient called an NIH surgeon at home, trying to get their patients or constituents to the head of the queue. We wanted the procedure to be fair to all candidates, not just to those with good political connections.

Question 6: What procedures will be employed to ensure that the consent of recipients or their families will be informed and voluntary? Achieving this goal was not easy with an approach to treatment as innovative as gene therapy. For severe combined immune deficiency, the families really needed a short course in immunology, and perhaps a second short course in the molecular biology of how vectors work.

Question 7: What steps will be taken to protect the privacy of gene therapy recipients and the confidentiality of medical information about them? The Human Gene Therapy Subcommittee did not want a replay of the circus-like atmosphere that had surrounded Barney Clark and his artificial heart, or Baby Faye and her transplanted baboon heart. We wanted patients and families to have space. I would like to compliment the press in this regard; they knew the family of Ashanti DeSilva from the time of her first treatment in 1990 and maintained the anonymity of the DeSilva family until the family was ready to go public.

The 'Points to Consider' document was not a philosopher's plot. But I should point out that one can array the seven questions I have just discussed under three principles of biomedical ethics that many of you have come to know and love (see Figure 3). These are principles from Tom Beauchamp and Jim Childress' book, *Principles of Biomedical Ethics*.[18] Beauchamp and Chil-

Ethical Principles and the "Points to Consider."

Beneficence
The disease and its natural history
Alternative therapies
Potential harms of the intervention
Potential benefits of the intervention

Justice
Selection of patient-subjects

Respect for Autonomy
Informed consent
Privacy and confidentiality

Figure 3.

dress themselves borrowed heavily from the National Commission for the Protection of Human Subjects.[19]

The questions about disease, alternative therapies, harms and benefits all fit under a principle Beauchamp and Childress call beneficence, which looks at harms, benefits, outcomes, consequences. In answering these questions, one can employ data from laboratory studies.

The question about fairness in the selection of patients is an illustration or an application of the principle of justice. It asks: How can harms or benefits be distributed in a fair or equitable manner?

The questions about voluntary and informed consent and privacy and confidentiality embody the third principle, respect for autonomy of persons.

You might say that these principles form a kind of a checklist. One can examine a protocol by asking these question or apply the questions to any new biomedical technology, just to make sure that one is looking at the protocol or technology from every side.

Just as important as these substantive questions was the fact that we had a transparent national public review process. Policy makers knew exactly what was going on. Any interested member of the public could attend a RAC meeting, see the investigators, hear what questions were being asked and have access to a public list of all the currently approved gene therapy protocols.

As of February 1998, 200 therapeutic gene-transfer protocols had been submitted to the National Institutes of Health and the Food and Drug Adminstration, 23 dealing with infectious disease (all of them HIV infection or AIDS), 33 dealing with single gene diseases (especially cystic fibrosis), 138 dealing with cancer, and six focused on other diseases. At the June 1998 RAC meeting, a first protocol for hemophilia A was presented, and a new kind of vector was proposed for the first time—a replication-competent herpes virus vector.

What lessons can we learn from these past 18 years? First, somatic cell gene therapy has been successfully distinguished from more ambitious plans for human genetic engineering. In that sense, some of the writings of the late 1970s, including writings by Jeremy Rifkin (for example, *Who Should Play God?*),[20] have been defeated in the public forum.

Somatic cell genetic intervention has been accepted by the public and by policy makers as analogous to bone marrow transplantation or organ transplantation, and not as the first step on a slippery slope toward the genetic engineering of the human race. In my view, it is an unmixed good that this distinction has been drawn.

Second, I sometimes wonder whether the wrong term was not chosen for the first 18 years of this potential, then actual biomedical intervention. Perhaps the term should have been human gene *transfer*, rather than human gene *therapy*. Why? If a researcher includes the phrase "human gene therapy" in the title of a protocol, that phrase seems to promise a benefit to the patient. There can be all kinds of provisos in the consent form, but once the notion of therapy is there, it is difficult to dismiss it from one's mind—especially if one is afflicted with a life-threatening disease.

"Human gene transfer" is a bit more neutral; the phrase describes what is actually happening. In virtually all of the protocols to date, the intent of the studies has been to be therapeutic. At the same time, however, there have been Phase-I studies whose main goal is to see whether a particular kind of human gene transfer is toxic to patients. Those studies were unlikely to be therapeutic for those particular patients.

Third, as I mentioned, a national public review process was established in the United States for research in this field. This model has been replicated in several other countries, albeit, in most cases, not with quite the same degree of publicity that the RAC has had in the United States, nor the same degree of public access to the process. The RAC structure and process may provide a helpful model for the future because there will be new issues coming down the pike. Xenotransplantation, transplants into humans from animals, is an issue right on the horizon. Perhaps germ line genetic intervention will be an issue at some point in the future, or even human embryo research. These all are kinds of activities that I think could benefit from a public advisory committee accountable to the public and policy makers, that could assure the public about what is going on in that particular field.

Each RAC-like review body could be established with a sunset clause; it would automatically cease to exist after perhaps five or ten years. A public advisory committee of this kind could help to introduce a new area of biomedical research; then perhaps the need for this group would disappear as the new approach either proved successful or failed. Had such a body been in place in the late 1960s, when cardiac transplants first began to be performed, I think we would have saved ourselves a great deal of grief, and many patients would have been spared premature death in poorly-designed surgical research.

A fourth conclusion: The success of human gene transfer has been quite modest in the first eight years. One can point to three or four studies and say yes, it does look as if new blood vessels have grown in the limbs of patients, or it does seem that Ashanti DeSilva and Cynthia Cutshall have been aided by a combination of gene therapy and a synthetic enzyme. Perhaps in a few chronic granulomatous disease patients there are some early signs of benefit. But the denominator for these few partial successes is the 200 protocols that had been developed and submitted by early 1998.

I regret to say that there have been times during the past eight years when researchers or companies have been guilty of overstating their early results. One of the roles of a public advisory committee is to be objective and sober and to demythologize this kind of exaggeration.

Fifth, the public review process for human gene transfer also revealed certain general deficiencies in the clinical research system in the United States. The Institutional Review Board (IRB) system, at times, seems not to have functioned well with gene transfer protocols. Poorly designed studies have been approved by local IRBs and passed on to the RAC for review. Consent forms have sometimes made it sound as though a Phase-I study will cure a patient's cancer.

We in the United States still have not bitten the bullet on what happens if patients, through no fault of the researchers, are injured while taking part in research on behalf of the whole society. The United Kingdom has a wonderful system in place, both for drug company-sponsored studies and for publicly funded studies. A highly-effective compensation system for all injuries to patients also exists in Sweden. We in the U.S. still cannot get our act together after 20 years of discussion and debate. If you want to see artful evasion, just look at the point in consent forms that describes what will happen if a subject is injured in the course of research.

Sixth and finally, I think we are having to face, right at the present moment, the question of what is the optimum location for any national public review body that looks at new biomedical technologies. I will put forward for your consideration the thesis that the National Institutes of Health (NIH) may not be the best location. NIH is the primary funding agency for biomedical research in the U.S. There may be times when an oversight function or an accountability function will come into conflict with the desire to do research as quickly and efficiently as possible.

Where else to go? The U.S. Food and Drug Administration (FDA) does much of its work in secret. Within the confidentiality policy of the FDA, the public does not generally know whether a study is beginning, when a study is beginning, or who is sponsoring in the study, so the FDA does not seem to be the proper agency either. Perhaps the review needs to be moved one level higher, to the level of the Department of Health and Human Services, or even to the level of the office of the President and the President's science advisor. Particularly in light of the conflict over the role of the RAC in the past two years, I think that one ought to reexamine whether NIH is the best place for the public oversight and public review of human gene transfer protocols in the U.S.

The next 18 years

What can we expect in the next 18 years? None of us really can see to the year 2016, but here are some things that I think are likely to happen.

In the somatic cell gene transfer arena, I think we will see studies that attempt to intervene at the prenatal stage to prevent damage to fetuses that would have been severe and irreversible by the time of birth. There have been a few in utero cell therapy studies approved by the FDA. There have been a few published results from these studies, including some reports of apparent successes. In addition, much work going on in this area in the laboratory, with animal models.

There is another area that I think will emerge: if you saw *the Scientific American* special feature on gene therapy in June of 1997, there was an entire article devoted to gene transfer for the prevention or treatment of neurological disease.[21] That will be a qualitatively new step for the field of somatic cell gene therapy—when Parkinson's disease or the deleterious effects of an accident or a stroke are treated by means of gene therapy. Thus far, most researchers have been cautious about trying to reach the brain because of the technical difficulties involved in delivering vectors and new genes into brain cells.

When we start to see studies affecting the brain, I think the question of what is enhancement and what is cure, treatment, or prevention of disease will arise in an acute form. For example, if one could intervene in such a way that a child destined to have an IQ of 60 or 70 would instead now have an IQ of 100, would one call the intervention remediation or enhancement?

Enhancement normally conveys the notion that someone is already in the normal range and is then given a boost above the normal range—like athletes taking performance-enhancing drugs in the effort to gain a competitive edge. But enhancement to bring someone who is below the normal range into the normal range may be the kind of enhancement that many of us would find morally justifiable.

In the next 18 years there also will be proposals for germ-line genetic intervention. A great deal of technical work will need to be done. Essentially, the breakthrough required will be a move away from the current technologies of gene addition, where a gene is put into cells in a such a way that it does not matter where the new DNA integrates; as long as it functions properly, it can do its job in the cell. (A close analogy is the 'insert' function of a word processor.)

In the future, what will be needed is something analogous to the global 'search and replace' function in word processing software—a program so sophisticated, a vector so clever, that it can find the malfunctioning gene, splice it out, and replace it with a properly functioning gene.

There are plausible moral arguments in favor of germ-line genetic intervention. It is more efficient than repeating somatic cell gene therapy, generation after generation. In one fell swoop, one could prevent, for example, cystic fibrosis, in all the future members of a particular family line, unless a new gene mutation were to arise later on.

Another argument is that, for some diseases, even in utero gene therapy is too late—the damage is done early in embryonic development or cannot be repaired after cell differentiation occurs. If we are going to try to cope with these diseases, rather than throwing up our hands in despair, we may have to intervene at the pre-implantation stage. Some families may be opposed in principle to pre-implantation diagnosis and selective discard. For those families, having an additional option could turn out to be quite important.

Finally, the one case that I have seen in the bioethics literature that seems to me to justify cloning, in the technical sense of nuclear transfer, is one that envisions a scenario in which a woman is likely to pass on mitochondrial disease to her offspring.[22] Most people think of cloning as confined to the time after birth—when somatic cells are removed from a child, an adult, or an older person. In the case that I am envisioning there would be nuclear transfer at the early embryonic stage. The scenario would go something like this. In vitro fertilization would be performed with sperm from the husband and an egg from the wife. At, say, the four-cell stage, the nuclei would be removed from all the embryonic cells and transferred into enucleated egg cells from a donor. (The mitochondria are in the cytoplasm of the cell.) In the new setting, if the intervention were successful, the embryos would be free from mitochondrial disease.

This is in fact a case that would simultaneously involve germ-line genetic intervention and cloning (in the technical sense of nuclear transfer). I do not know where we will come out in our ethical evaluation of this kind of proposal, but I think that it present the most plausible (and the most health-related) case for the moral justifiability of cloning, in the technical sense.

What should be the goals of germ-line genetic intervention? In general, I think, the goals should be to prevent or alleviate disease and disability.

Gene therapy and eugenics

In conclusion, I would like to compare and contrast current somatic cell gene therapy and possible future proposals for germ-line genetic intervention with a very sad chapter in human history, namely the mandatory eugenics programs in the United States and the German Reich in the first half of this century. I do not mean to be unfair to researchers in making this comparison; In my view, human gene transfer research has generally been conducted in a highly responsible way. But a look at this sad history may help us to see certain features, certain differences, and certain grounds for our concern about the future of genetic intervention.

Here is the Virginia statute for eugenic sterilization from 1924:

> Whereas, human experience has demonstrated that heredity plays an important part in the transmission of insanity, idiocy, imbecility, epilepsy and crime, now therefore: Be it enacted by the General Assembly of Virginia, that whenever the superintendent [of one of the four state hospitals] shall be of the opinion... and so forth... sterilization can be performed on anyone [who is] afflicted with hereditary forms of insanity that are recurrent, idiocy, imbecility, feeble-mindedness or epilepsy; provided that such superintendent shall have first complied with the requirements of this act.[23]

Why feature the statute from Virginia? In 1927, the United States Supreme Court decided the case *Buck v. Bell*.[24] Oliver Wendell Holmes wrote the majority decision that found this statute to be constitutional. To his decision Holmes appended the infamous line: "Three generations of imbeciles are enough."

Here is a second statute—from July 14, 1933, from the German Reich. The translation comes from Burleigh and Wipperman's book, *The Racial State*:

> Anyone who has a hereditary illness can be rendered sterile by a surgical operation, if according to the experience of medical science, there is a strong probability that his/her progeny will suffer from serious hereditary defect of a physical or mental nature. Anyone is hereditarily ill within the meaning of the new law who suffers from one of the following illnesses.[25]

Here are the eight kinds of illnesses that made people liable to appear before the genetic courts in Germany in the late 1930s: congenital feeble-mindedness, schizophrenia, manic depression, hereditary epilepsy, Huntington's chorea, hereditary blindness, hereditary deafness, serious physical deformities. And then almost as an afterthought, the sterilization statute added a ninth category: "Anyone who suffers from chronic alcoholism can be sterilized."

From what sources did the National Socialists derive the inhumane and discriminatory categories for their sterilization statute? One can find the intellectual roots in a book that an American, Harry Laughlin, published in 1922,

Eugenical Sterilization in the United States.[26] The German list is taken almost verbatim from a list in Harry Laughlin's book.

In fact, one might even say that the National Socialists were a bit more differentiated, slightly more scientific than Harry Laughlin. They deliberately omitted one of Laughlin's groups of people who could be sterilized, the "dependent (including orphans, ne'er-do-wells, the homeless, tramps and paupers)."[27]

There were advocates for the reform and control of the excesses of the eugenic sterilization movement in the United States already in the 1920s. Here I would like to pay tribute to a wonderful neurologist and psychiatrist, Abraham Myerson. Myerson, was born into a Jewish family in the ghetto village of Yanova, Lithuania, in 1881. When Abraham was five years old, his father, Morris Myerson, brought the family to the United States. After growing to adulthood and completing his medical training and residency, Abraham settled in Boston where he taught at Tufts University Medical Center and had a private practice in neurology and psychiatry.[28] In 1925, he published a book, *The Inheritance of Mental Diseases*,[29] which should have been required reading for the justices of the U.S. Supreme Court and especially for Oliver Wendell Holmes. In that book, Myerson surveyed what was known at the time about the inheritance of various kinds of mental disease and cut the props out from under much of the eugenics rubbish that was being foisted on the American public at the time.[30]

In 1936 Myerson and a committee of the American Neurological Association published a review of sterilization, in which they concluded that sterilization programs should be strictly voluntary, either for the person involved or for persons making decisions about their children or their wards.[31] But this group, too, had a list in descending order of importance and justifiability. In 1936, they said that eugenic sterilization could be undertaken for (1) people with (a) Huntington's chorea; (b) hereditary optic atrophy—a disease that destroys the optic nerve and causes impairment of vision; (c) familial cases of Friedreich's ataxia, a disease that causes unsteady gait, then paralysis, and then contractures; and (d) "certain other disabling degenerative diseases recognized to be hereditary."[32]

Continuing down the list, the American Neurological Association also recommended that selective sterilization be considered for: (2) feeble-mindedness of familial type; (3) schizophrenia; (4) manic depressive psychosis; and (5) epilepsy.[33] Thus, I am sad to say, even some of the most enlightened critics of eugenic sterilization had their own list of conditions that could justify this invasive intervention.

How do the diseases on these lists compare with the diseases that have been targeted for human gene therapy thus far? If one were drawing a Venn diagram, there would be virtually no overlap. In the one circle we have cancer, severe combined immune deficiency, HIV infection and AIDS (which were not even around in the 1920s and 1930s), and vascular disorders of various types. But as we move to the next stage, and particularly as somatic cell genetic intervention starts to deal with brain diseases, we will be returning to territory that is closer to the concerns of the eugenics movement in the early 20th century.

Thus, somatic cell gene therapy is totally different from eugenic sterilization in the sense that eugenic sterilization aimed to cut something off in the germ-line, whereas somatic cell human gene transfer aims only to help a particular patient. But as we move, as I think we will, to germ-line intervention, the question of hereditary transmission will recur. It is because of these earlier instances of vicious and destructive intervention in the germ-line that many people are so uneasy about germ-line genetic intervention, even for the noble purpose of trying to prevent or cure disease. Especially in continental Europe, there is a widely shared skepticism about any kind of germ-line genetic intervention.

Notice that in each generation we develop new terms, new concepts to describe diseases and disabilities. None of us talks about "idiocy" or "imbecility" anymore. Phrases like "intellectual disability" and "people with mental retardation" are much more respectful. We have to be open to the fact that 50 years from now our disease categories and classifications may turn out to have been just as misguided as those earlier classifications were.

We should note, also, that how serious a disease or disability is thought to be varies over time. Think about people with visual impairment, people with hearing impairment, people with epilepsy, and people with bipolar affective disorder. In all of these cases we look at persons affected by these disabilities or disorders in a totally different way. In fact, the Americans with Disabilities Act of 1990 embodies the notion that we should maximize what people with some of these handicaps can do in the workplace and in their lives. In criticizing the past, we should also remember that new therapies can have an effect on how we view certain disorders. Epilepsy, if it led to repeated seizures every day, would be one disease; epilepsy controlled by medication is quite a different disorder.

The groups enumerated in the three lists cited above have been stigmatized and victimized in the past. The degree of victimization varied. In Virginia, sterilization was the price of freedom from lifetime incarceration for the intellectually disabled. This coercive sterilization process for so-called imbeciles was upheld as constitutional by a near-unanimous vote of the U.S. Supreme Court. The sterilization program in Nazi Germany, which involved hundreds of thousands of people, was followed by an extermination program directed first toward children, then toward adults who were mentally ill or intellectually impaired. And even the reform-minded proposals of Abraham Myerson's committee encouraged specific groups to accept sterilization for themselves or to have their children sterilized.

What, then, should we do? First, everyone interested in human genetics needs to take a stand and to say *never again*—never again genetic discrimination, whether it be in gene hunting, genetic testing, or attempts to perform gene transfer. This challenge applies both to professionals and to members of the public. Never again will we allow people with Huntington's disease, or intellectual disabilities, or visual impairment to be treated with disrespect.

There is an inevitable tension here. We can applaud the war on disease that genetic research is waging. It will be a great day when a child is definitively cured of cystic fibrosis or when a particular family line is liberated from the burden of fragile-X syndrome. But we will be humane warriors only if, in the midst of the battle, we also manifest our care for those who courageously cope with disability and for those who cannot yet be cured.

Acknowledgment

Substantial portions of this presentation were also given at the conference on "The Human Genome Project: Science, Law, and Social Change in the 21st Century" sponsored by the Whitehead Institute for Biomedical Research in Cambridge, Massachusetts, on April 23rd and 24th, 1998. The author wishes to thank the Whitehead Institute for permission to reprint some of his earlier remarks.

Notes

1. Demaret, 1984, pp. 120–124.
2. For a fuller account of David's story, see Walters, Palmer, 1997, pp. xiii–xviii.
3. Shearer, et al., 1985, pp. 1151–1159.
4. *Time*, 1993, pp. 50–53.
5. For the text of this letter, see President's Commission for the Study of Ethical Problems in Medicine and Biomedical and Behavioral Research, 1982, pp. 95–96.
6. Jacobs, 1980, pp. 1, 26.
7. Anderson, Fletcher, 1980, pp. 1293–1297.
8. Parliamentary Assembly, Council of Europe, 1982.
9. See note 5 above.
10. United States, Congress, Office of Technology Assessment, 1984.
11. National Institutes of Health, Recombinant DNA Advisory Committee, 1985.
12. Nichols, Institute of Medicine, National Academy of Sciences, 1988.
13. For a fuller account of the work of the RAC during the early years of gene therapy, see Walters, Palmer, 1997, Chapter 5 (see note 2 above).
14. The executive summary of the Verma Committee report from September 8, 1995, is available at the following URL: www.nih.gov/od/oba.
15. See Marshall, 1995, p. 1751. The full text of the Orkin-Motulsky committee report is available at the following URL: www.nih.gov/od/oba.
16. Up-to-date protocol lists can be viewed at the following URL: www.nih.gov/od/oba.

17. The current version of the "Points to Consider" is included in Appendix M of the NIH Guidelines for Recombinant DNA Research. See the following URL: www.nih.gov/od/oba.
18. Beauchamp, Childress, 1994.
19. National Commission for the Protection of Human Subjects, 1979, pp. 23192–23197.
20. Howard, Rifkin, 1977.
21. Ho, Sapolsky, 1997, pp. 116–120.
22. Rubinstein et al., 1995, pp. 316–339.
23. Quoted from Lombardo, 1982, p. 268.
24. *United States [Supreme Court] Reports* 274 (1927), pp. 200–208.
25. Burleigh, Wippermann, 1991, p. 137.
26. Laughlin, *Eugenical Sterilization in the United States* (Chicago: Psychopathic Laboratory of the Municipal Court of Chicago, December 1922), pp. 446–447.
27. Ibid., p. 447.
28. This biographical sketch is based on Mildred Ann Myerson's "Abraham Myerson: A Biographical Note," in Abraham Myerson, Speaking of Man, 1950, pp. 253–276.
29. Myerson, 1925.
30. See especially Myerson, 1925, pp. 13, 64–67,73–83.
31. Myerson, et al., 1936.
32. Ibid., p. 179.
33. Ibid.

Bibliography

Anderson, W. F., Fletcher, J. C. 1980. "Gene Therapy in Humans: When Is It Ethical to Begin?" *New England Journal of Medicine* 303, 22, pp. 1293–1297

Beauchamp, T. L., Childress, J. F., 1994. *Principles of Biomedical Ethics* (4th ed.). Oxford University Press: New York.

Burleigh, M., Wippermann, W., 1991. *The Racial State: Germany 1933–1945*. Cambridge University Press: Cambridge.

Demaret, K. 1984. "David's Story." *People Weekly*, October 29, pp. 120–124.

Laughlin, H. H., 1922. *Eugenical Sterilization in the United States*. Psychopathic Laboratory of the Municipal Court of Chicago: Chicago.

Ho, D. Y., Sapolsky, R. M., 1997. "Gene Therapy for the Nervous System." *Scientific American* 276, 6, pp. 116–120.

Howard, T., Rifkin, J., 1977. *Who Should Play God?* Dell Publishing Company: New York.

Jacobs, P., 1980. "Pioneer Genetic Implants Revealed." *Los Angeles Times*, 8 October, pp. 1, 26.

Lombardo, P.A., 1982. "Eugenic Sterilization in Virginia: Aubrey Strode and the Case of Buck v. Bell.", Appendix B. Unpublished Ph.D. dissertation. University of Virginia.

Marshall, E. "Less Hype, More Biology Needed for Gene Therapy." *Science* 70, 5243, p. 1751

Myerson, A., 1925. *The Inheritance of Mental Diseases*. Williams and Wilkins: Baltimore.

Myerson, A. et al., American Neurological Association, Committee for the Investigation of Eugenical Sterilization, 1936. *Eugenical Sterilization: A Reorientation of the Problem*. Macmillan: New York.

Myerson, M. A. 1950. "Abraham Myerson: A Biographical Note." In: Myerson, A. *Speaking of Man*. Alfred A. Knopf: New York, pp. 253–276.

National Commission for the Protection of Human Subjects, 1979. "Protection of Human Subjects: Belmont Report: Ethical Principles and Guidelines for the Protection of Human Subjects of Research..." *Federal Register* 44, 76, pp. 23192–23197.

National Institutes of Health, Recombinant DNA Advisory Committee, 1985. "Recombinant DNA Research : Request for Public Comment on 'Points to Consider in the Design and Submission of Human Somatic-Cell Gene Therapy Protocols.'" *Federal Register* 50, 14, pp. 2940–2945.

Nichols, E. K., Institute of Medicine, National Academy of Sciences, 1988. *Human Gene Therapy.* Harvard University Press: Cambridge.

Parliamentary Assembly, Council of Europe, 1982. "Recommendation 934 (1982) on Genetic Engineering." In: *Texts Adopted by the Assembly*, 33rd Ordinary Session, Third Part, January 25–29, Strasbourg.

President's Commission for the Study of Ethical Problems in Medicine and Biomedical and Behavioral Research, 1982. *Splicing Life*. Appendix B. Government Printing Office: Washington D.C., pp. 95–96.

Rubinstein, D.S. et al., 1995. "Germ-Line Therapy to Cure Mitochondrial Disease: Protocol and Ethics of *in vitro* Ovum Nuclear Transfer." *Cambridge Quarterly of Healthcare Ethics* 4, 3, pp. 316–339.

Shearer, W. T. et al.,1985. "Epstein-Barr Virus-Associated B-Cell Proliferations of Diverse Clonal Origins after Bone Marrow Transplantation in a 12-Year-Old Patient with Severe Combined Immunodeficiency." *New England Journal of Medicine* 312, 18, pp. 1151–1159.

Time, 7 June 1993, pp. 50–53.

United States, Congress, Office of Technology Assessment, 1984. *Human Gene Therapy: Background Paper.* OTA December 1984, Washington D.C.

United States [Supreme Court] Reports. Vol. 274, 1927, pp. 200–208.

Walters, L., Palmer, J. G., 1997. *The Ethics of Human Gene Therapy.* Oxford University Press: New York.

CHARLES WEINER

Social Responsibility in Genetic Engineering: Historical Perspectives

What are the ethical limits to human genetic intervention? This question should be high on the public agenda as we enter the twenty first century. New technologies, pervasive commercialization, and extraordinary claims by researchers, funding agencies and entrepreneurs provide relentless pressure to continuously shift the line of ethically acceptable applications of human genetic engineering. The policy decisions that must be made require full public participation and should take into account societal values, relevant technical information and the cumulative experience gained from past efforts to anticipate and control the consequences of the uses of genetic knowledge. I will provide several historical perspectives on these issues to reveal patterns that may be useful in understanding the present. My focus is on how scientists in the field have dealt with the ethical, social and political consequences of genetic engineering.

Social responsibility in science

The concept of social responsibility and accountability of scientists took on a special meaning after the atomic bombs were dropped on Hiroshima and Nagasaki in 1945. Individually, and in organizations formed around issues such as arms control, many scientists in the postwar decades saw the need to exercise responsibility in their research and its applications. They wanted to avoid doing harm and to prevent abuse of research results. This included examining the context in which scientific work is done, anticipating negative or unintended consequences, and refusing to participate in projects deemed to be socially harmful. Concerned scientists also felt the need to provide early warning to colleagues and to the larger society and to provide information to the public by speaking out publically.

Social accountability was especially important for biologists because of the relevance of their work to life, health, and the environment. For example, in the postwar decades many biologists campaigned against biological warfare research emphasizing that they were committed to the life sciences and the improvement of health, not to "death" science which caused destruction and disease.[1]

Genetic engineering and ethics in the 1960s and 70s

Rapid progress in genetics in the 1950s and 1960s, including the discovery of the double helix structure of DNA and the unraveling of the genetic code, raised expectations about the ability to understand life processes at a fundamental level and to eventually apply this knowledge to the manipulation of genes. Biologists' excitement about these prospects was often accompanied by concern about the political, social and ethical implications of the new genetics.

The message was strongly stated by one of the first distinguished scientists to speak out, the president of the Nobel Foundation, Swedish biochemist Arne Tiselius who was a professor at the University of Uppsala and had received the Nobel Prize in 1948 for his work on electrophoresis. In 1961, on the occasion of the 60th anniversary of the prize, Tiselius spoke about the moral obligations of scientists in the applications of their work in weapons of mass destruction and also in "the search into the very basis of the life process." He said that "it is possible—many think even probable—" that the new biological research "will lead to methods of tampering with life, of creating new diseases, of controlling the psyche, of influencing heredity, even perhaps in certain desired directions." He warned that this could "result in a still more refined and perhaps still more dangerous way of abusing the results of research than that implied in the instruments of mass destruction." Tiselius argued that because of this prospect "we see the demand for an international moral code governing the use of scientific results as a self-evident necessity."[2]

Subsequent discussions among biologists in the 1960s focused on when and where to draw the line in the applications of human genetic engineering. This was an anticipatory concern since recombinant DNA and related genetic manipulation techniques were not available at that time. Discussion at scientific meetings of the prospects for human genetic intervention and its ethical limits soon reached the media and the political process and some biologists feared that public "overreaction" would interfere with their research interests and their funding. They tried to reassure the public that the work would be beneficial or that it was too early to worry about negative effects. Others argued that the ethical consequences of genetic engineering should be anticipated and discussed in advance, before it was too late as in the case of the atomic bomb. This was very vivid imagery. It is worth looking at in some detail, because of its relevance to our current discussions.[3]

In January 1962, a few months after Tiselius' statement, a *New York Times* editorial, "The Code of Life", observed that the recent deciphering of an important part of the genetic code could lead to "a revolution far greater in its potential significance than the atomic or hydrogen bomb." Quoting Tiselius' warning, the editorial concluded that "It is not too soon to be prepared against such potential abuses."[4]

In 1963, the *Times* made an editorial comment on the 11th International Congress of Genetics which had just concluded in Europe:

> Geneticists are on the threshold of a historic breakthrough in their efforts to probe the secrets of heredity... Is mankind ready for such powers? The moral, economic and political implications of these possibilities are staggering, yet they have received little. . . organized public consideration. The danger exists that the scientists will make some of these God-like powers available to us in the next few years well before society—on present evidence—is likely to be even remotely prepared for the ethical and other dilemmas with which we shall be faced.[5]

The appropriate time and place for discussing ethical consequences was also an issue at a small private meeting of leading biologists held at Rockefeller University in 1966. The invitation to the meeting reviewed work being carried out in several laboratories that seemed promising for human genetic engineering, noting that "the problem is obviously immense and almost fantastic in implication. Unless a massive frontal assault is made, it will be many years before something that could be accomplished in the foreseeable future will be achieved." The intention was to set up a committee "to discuss and program what could and should be done and after deciding this and its cost to get support and hire the proper scientists."[6] The minutes of the meeting reveal the participants' views on the advent of genetic engineering, and their reluctance to discuss it publicly.

After discussing how to build and test genetic material, the participants asked: "Do we use it?" Their answer was that if such reagents were made they would "be used whether we like it or not. What can be done, is done, and what can be used, is used. The main variable is the rate of development and application. Proper use depends on active supervision by interested persons who are involved in the original accomplishment."

Then they discussed whether they should stimulate anything of this kind, asking if any step would be an escalation. They concluded that "if it is not done by us, others will do it and they won't do it as well." They also pondered whether they could discuss the feasibility of such endeavors without discussing the desirability. One participant noted that eugenic potential had been available for many years and had not been used. Another noted that "eugenic measures generally have negative elements which involve large social structures and are therefore resisted while genetic intervention is mostly positive and on an individual basis and as such has qualities analogous to those which sell soap."

The participants decided that there would be no publication of their discussion nor an official report. They felt that " there is too little in the way of hard materials," and that "this area is so highly charged that no matter how carefully anything is said, it gets overplayed and over-interpreted".[7] Their decision to control the information and keep it from the public was paternalistic and unrealistic since the research was publically funded (as was their meeting) and the possible applications to human genetic engineering clearly were of public concern. The prospect of genetic engineering was already public, and it continued to be. Eight months later in an editorial in *Science* magazine, Marshall Nirenberg, the biologist whose work on the genetic code had contributed one of the important steps to the new genetic revolution, and who was to win a Nobel Prize in 1968, took a different position:

> Man may be able to program his own cells with synthetic information long before he'll be able to assess adequately the long-term consequences of such alterations, long before he'll be able to formulate goals and long before he can resolve the ethical and moral problems which will be raised. When man becomes capable of instructing his own cells, he must refrain from doing so until he has sufficient wisdom to use this knowledge for the benefit of mankind. I state this problem well in advance of the need to resolve it because decisions concerning the application of this knowledge must ultimately be made by society and only an informed society can make such decisions wisely.[8]

The new developments in genetics were also discussed publicly by the geneticist Joshua Lederberg in a series of columns in *The Washington Post*. The Nobel Laureate's reassuring views were challenged by Leon Kass, a young biologist at the National Institutes of Health, who had organized a bioethics seminar there. He responded in the *Post* in November 1967:

> The possibility of genetic manipulation in man raises fundamental and enormous questions, theological, moral, political. These questions must be carefully stated, the issues clearly articulated and the alternative policies fully and soberly considered... The development of science and technology, once begun, often proceeds without deliberated and considered decisions. Considerations of desirability rarely govern the transition from "it can be done" to "it has been done." Biologists today are under strong obligation to raise just such questions publicly so that we may deliberate *before* the new biomedical technology is an accomplished fact, a technology whose consequences will probably dwarf those which resulted from the development of the atomic bomb.[9]

In 1969 Jonathan Beckwith, a young molecular geneticist at Harvard Medical School, and his colleagues held a remarkable press conference to announce that they had achieved the first purification and isolation of a bacterial gene, a significant step in the direction of genetic engineering. Their purpose was not to seek acclaim for their results but to sound the alarm about the possible negative social and political consequences of manipulating genes.[10] The popular press response included headlines about "genetic bombs", and the scientific press vehemently criticized the researchers' actions as irresponsible behavior that might cause a threat to scientific funding. Beckwith and his colleagues responded in a letter to the journal *Nature*:

> As we see it, scientists are obligated to inform the public about what is happening in their secluded fields of research so that people can demand control over decisions which profoundly affect their lives. If our arguments mean [as our critics say] that "the progress of science itself may be interrupted," that is an unfortunate consequence we will have to accept. It certainly should not inhibit us from speaking out on crucial issues.[11]

Several months later, in April 1970, when he received the prestigious Ely Lilly Award for his work, Beckwith included a political critique and plea for social responsibility in his acceptance address entitled "Gene Expression in Bacteria and Some Concerns About the Misuse of Science."[12] In the decades since then he has continued his research while acting on his sense of social responsibility in critiques and studies of abuses of genetic screening, the use of genetics to promulgate eugenic and racist policies, and the growing tendency to overemphasize the role of genetics in disease and social problems.[13] He persisted despite resistance from the professional structures of science, and received recognition for this integrated role in 1993 when the Genetics Society of America awarded him their Medal for both his science and his social policy role.

Biologists' concerns about where and when to draw the line in genetic engineering were highlighted in a 1970 London conference on "The Social Impact of Modern Biology." The speakers included leading biologists and many nonscientists were in the audience of more than 800. In one discussion, a geneticist argued:

> We are just deluding ourselves if we think that human genetic engineering is so in the realm of science fiction that we don't need to start thinking about it. My worry is that the advances will be extremely slow and minor to begin with. For instance, I would estimate that within four or five years it will be possible to cure, to a very minor, limited extent, by genetic engineering, certain genetic deficiencies. Nobody will object to that. And so we will go on to the next step, and the next step, and so on. If we don't start discussing these matters now we shall get to the state as we did with the atom bomb, when nobody knows what is going on.[14]

The continuing emphasis was that prior discussion provided time to think about the issues, before technological momentum builds up and applications are imminent, and before vested interests take over. The symbol of the mushroom cloud was intertwined with the symbol of the double helix.

Specific concern about the claims being made for gene therapy were expressed in July 1971 by two geneticists, Maurice Fox of MIT and John Littlefield of Harvard, in a *Science* guest editorial entitled "Reservations Concerning Gene Therapy". They called for a realistic appraisal of its potential and a sober consideration of its liabilities. They cautioned that many of the procedures were likely to be mutagenic and that many dominant effects visible only in the whole individual might appear. They noted that most of the viruses under consideration as vectors were tumor-producing and that "damaging alterations of regulatory processes and even uncontrolled tumor-like growth could easily be the consequences of introducing additional chromosomes or a host of viral genes." Fox and Littlefield concluded:

> The promises offered by the proponents of gene therapy largely ignore its limitations and hazards. To mislead the public in this regard risks another period of disappointment and reaction. We are still primarily in a descriptive phase in our understanding of human genetics, with little, if any, idea of how to intervene safely at any level. Let us not do to ourselves what we have done to our environment. Let us now seek public support for research for better understanding of normal and abnormal human biology, rather than promise quick glamorous cures.[15]

One other example of this early concern is the 1972 statement by French Anderson who has consistently pushed the limits of acceptance of gene therapy since then: "The potential uses and misuses of genetic intervention are so great that now is the time to examine closely what is being done and where it may lead. Society does not want to learn of the consequences of a scientific accomplishment only after great damage has already been inflicted, as was the case with nuclear power."[16]

There are many more examples of the anticipatory interest in the ethical problems of genetic intervention that was expressed within the international community of biologists in the pre-recombinant DNA period. But things began to change when public interest in the subject increased, culminating in the United States with congressional hearings in the late 1960s to consider the need for a national commission on health, science, and society. The purpose: to anticipate, to examine in advance, and to report on the legal, ethical and social implications of biomedical research, including genetic engineering. It was meant to be a study commission, without the intention of interfering with research. The focus was on new, emerging, medical technologies such as the artificial heart, organ transplants, new reproductive technologies, and also genetic engineering, which was not possible at the time, but on the horizon.

Although some of the biologists who participated in the hearings showed genuine concern about the issues raised, others feared that their funding might be cut off or severely curtailed and were defensive about the nature and usefulness of their work. They worried about what they perceived as public intervention in the scientific process and the possibility of loss of control. Several of them tried to reassure the public by arguing that concerns about human genetic intervention were premature and that it was too early to deal with them. Some pointed to several immediate, visible problems arising from new medical interventions, and maintained that they were more worthy of concern than "the more lurid speculations" about the future applications of genetics. They argued that government intervention would stop progress and delay cures for dread diseases, and that more funds were needed for beneficial research.[17]

While the efforts to anticipate and study the ethical and social implications of genetic engineering faded, the new recombinant DNA techniques were being developed. In 1970 a planned experiment at Paul Berg's Stanford laboratory would have introduced the SV40 tumor virus into a bacterium as a step in developing tools for genetic manipulation. When scientists at Cold Spring Harbor learned of this they were alarmed about the possible safety hazards of the work and urged Berg to abandon the experiment. Berg postponed it and sought other alternatives. The focus was on the biohazard problem, not on the larger ethical implications of genetic engineering. A notable exception was the effort by Leon Kass to raise the ethical issues with Berg in a dinner conversation followed up by a long letter to him in October 1970. This remarkable document outlined questions of efficacy and safety, limits to uses, possible undesirable consequences, and monitoring and control of human genetic manipulation.[18] But these concerns were submerged in the subsequent efforts to develop the technical tools for manipulating genes.

At the Gordon Conference on Nucleic Acids in July 1973, scientists revealed startling results using the newly discovered restriction enzymes to cut strands of DNA at precise points, to combine them with the DNA of other organisms and even other species, and to clone myriad copies of this recombinant or hybrid DNA. Participants expressed concern about the possible implications of the work, but that concern was limited to the possibility of immediate laboratory safety hazards associated with the research being launched. They were worried that recombinant DNA experiments could unintentionally create human pathogens through the introduction of antibiotic resistance, that the work might produce dangerous toxins, and that it might transform benign materials into cancer-causing agents. In November 1974, during the six-month period when a temporary moratorium was invoked by the scientists in the field on those particular experiments thought to be potentially hazardous, two university biologists in California applied for a patent on the recombinant DNA technique. Thus, the age of genetic engineering was underway with the commercial applications protected and discussion of the ethical implications postponed.

The February 1975 Asilomar Conference brought together scientists in the field to consider the hazards of recombinant DNA research and to find ways to reduce them. In his opening remarks at the Asilomar Conference, David Baltimore expressed the views of the meeting's organizers:

> Although I think it's obvious that this technology is possibly the most potent potential technology in biological warfare, this meeting is not designed to deal with that question. The issue that does bring us here is that a new technique of molecular biology appears to have allowed us to outdo the standard events of evolution by making combinations of genes which could be immediate natural history. These pose special potential hazards while they offer enormous benefits. We are here in a sense to balance the benefits and hazards right now and to design a strategy which will maximize the benefits and minimize the hazards for the future.[19]

Their concerns were narrowed to the immediate technical problems of laboratory safety, and they developed technical solutions to these problems. During the political controversy in the mid 1970s about whether these "tech fixes" were adequate, leading scientists in the field argued that the imminent practical benefits of the research and the absence of demonstrated risk meant that it was imperative that the research proceed as rapidly as possible. Public expectations of valued benefits were raised while possible hazards were downplayed. Ethical issues related to the potential applications of the new research tools and techniques were largely ignored. *They focused on the means, not the ends.*

Commercialization in the 1980s

Recombinant DNA techniques had an enormous scientific and social impact. They made possible new basic research on the structure and function of genes, opened up new fields of inquiry and led to a variety of applications in industry, agriculture, and medicine. Biology has been transformed and so have been the biologists. Starting very rapidly in the early 1980s, academic biologists never before involved with industry became consultants, advisors, founders, equity holders, and contractees of new biotechnology firms or new divisions of multinational corporations. Current disputes over patents on DNA sequences, human cells, tissues and body parts, and experimental processes and products are prominent in the scientific and public media. New companies are continuing to form around the developing technologies in agriculture, pharmacology, gene sequencing, genetic testing, DNA profiling, and human gene therapy. Universities are aggressively setting up companies and cutting multi million dollar deals with industry.

The rapid, large scale commercialization of academic biology has created conflicts of interest that may seriously erode public trust. Now more than ever biologists' expert advice is urgently needed on questions of public policy. But the commercial roles and possible conflicts of interest of many biologists and their institutions have influenced their perceptions and their willingness to speak out, and limited their effectiveness as credible public advisors.

The Uppsala Code of Ethics from 1984

Before turning to the past decade, let us return to Sweden and Uppsala where Tiselius worked. As I noted earlier, his strong and prestigious voice in 1961 was one of the first to call attention to the potential power and possibilities of abuse of the new biology and he argued for establishment of a moral code for scientists. Twenty years later, in 1981, a new generation of scholars at Uppsala University began to study and discuss research ethics focusing on the responsibility of scientists for applications of their results. In 1984, the same year that the Swedish Gene Ethics committee issued its report on Genetic Integrity, the Code of Ethics for Scientists was published by the Uppsala group. It calls on scientists to assess the practical consequences of their research and to discontinue ethically doubtful research and inform others about this decision. The emphasis is on ecology and war, but it is meant to apply to all fields including biomedicine.[20] The Code was widely discussed in Sweden and stimulated continued thinking about these issues. In 1989 two of the participants in the group that formulated the Code offered an important observation: "the existence of ethical discussions and rules may be used to legitimate activities rather than to change them."[21] This warning has special relevance to the current approach to ethics in the human genome projects and discussions about human gene transfer.

Genetics and ethics today

How does the Human Genome Project's approach to ethical issues differ from the past? Although there are many similarities, one apparent difference is that the Project is making an effort to identify the ethical, legal and social issues in advance, preparing society to deal with the "non-beneficial" uses of the vast amount of genetic information the project is designed to produce. But if this effort is compartmentalized and insulated from the main mission of the project without influencing its policies and priorities, then it once again separates the technical from the ethical, and defers the ethical issues, defining them as a societal and not a scientific concern. George Annas observed in 1989 that "ethics is generally taken seriously by physicians and scientists only when it either fosters their agenda or does not interfere with it. If it cautions a slower pace or a more deliberate consideration of science's darker side, it is dismissed as 'fearful of the future,' anti-intellectual, or simply uninformed."[22] Fortunately there are some notable exceptions to this criticism.

Many scientists feel frustrated in approaching the issues. Witness, for example, a biologist's response to my question about the meager amount of discussion of ethical issues at a small conference he attended at Cold Spring Harbor in the early 1980s on the prospects for human gene therapy. He answered:

> I wanted more discussion on it... I did, and I didn't. There's a sense in which it's more fun to talk about the science. You're actually doing things in science. . . I think everyone who lived through the Asilomar period in the late 1970s and the regulatory period came to recognize that at the end of the day, when you're working with scientific things, you're in control. You, yourself, are in control of what you're doing, of your laboratory, or of your scientific environment in advance. When you get involved in regulatory, ethical, or political issues, you have to share that control and often you have very little input into what happens. I think that scientists like being in control. I think all of us find such situations at best ambiguous and at worst profoundly unsettling.[23]

Control over discussions, actions and policy in human genetic engineering has been a central issue in the past and continues into the present. When I interviewed biologists in the late 1970s about their roles in the recombinant DNA safety controversy, I also asked some of them for their views about limits to genetic manipulation. They felt that the line should be drawn before human gene therapy and that the ethical issues were too important to be decided by the scientists involved. They said that the society as a whole should decide whether to undertake human somatic cell therapy, and volunteered that they were personally opposed to germ line interventions. These were private, not public, statements. Soon after, the scientists in the field and their academic institutions and funding agencies were involved in the pervasive commercialization of biotechnology and genetic engineering. Despite government committees and commissions and the involvement of bioethicists, the marketplace is a major force today in national policies or lack of policies in gene therapy.

Discussions of informed consent, safety, patients' rights and other standard biomedical ethics topics seem to take place under the assumption that human gene therapy is inevitable. Instead of "just say no", it has become "do it right."[24] The focus of scientists in the field and of many bioethicists is not about drawing the line, but about shifting the line—from somatic cell interventions to germ line, from germ line to its components, medical and enhancement. The germ line taboo is giving way to campaigns for gaining public acceptance, otherwise known as "marketing." Today's approach brings to mind the statement from the minutes of the 1966 private meeting to explore human genetic engineering that I quoted earlier: "Genetic intervention... has qualities analogous to those which sell soap."

Today, some academic scientists and the companies they are affiliated with publicize genetic engineering research that they fear might be resisted on ethical grounds. Their motive seems to be to get the ethicists' blessings and the public's approval or acquiescence. They talk of potential benefits, the need to initiate public debate, and their conviction that "rational" decisions will be made. A current example is the claim of a U.S. company that it had made human cells revert to the embryonic state by fusing them with cow eggs to create a hybrid cell. The company scientist said that he was making the technique public now "because I want to be very open and level with everyone. We need to get the ethicists to talk about it so as to encourage a rational response to these new technologies... Any technology can be abused, but once the public understands how these cells can be used to treat any disease caused by loss or malfunction of cells, from Parkinson's to diabetes to heart disease, the concerns will be overshadowed."[25]

Another example is the conference at the University of California-Los Angeles in March 1998, proclaimed by its organizers as "the opening of the public debate about germ line therapy." Their intended outcome was clear when they went on to say that the conference would focus on "how , why and when germ line engineering should proceed." Eight of the ten speakers were prominent scientists, all advocating human germ line intervention, and the two non-scientists were not in opposition. The list of the scientists' prestigious scientific affiliations, prizes and editorships of key journals omitted their commercial involvements in biotechnology firms.

What did they have to say? You can take your pick from the newspaper and magazine accounts of this well publicized meeting or consult the proceedings themselves on the website [www.ess.ucla.edu/huge] set up by the organizers. Here are a few quotes from the proceedings that are especially interesting.

> French Anderson: "The unfortunate fact is that, with the exception of a few anecdotal cases, there is no evidence of a gene therapy protocol that helps in any disease situation."

If that is the case why persist in referring to these attempts as gene "therapy"? Gene transfer might be a better term, and less misleading.

> James Watson: "If we could make better human beings by knowing how to add genes, why shouldn't we do it?..." and at another point, "If you could cure a very serious disease, *stupidity*, that would be a great thing for the people who otherwise would be born seriously disadvantaged."

Leroy Hood noted that it will be "only a matter of time" before the results of the Human Genome Project are used in germline engineering to enhance the human species. Several of the speakers rejoiced in their claim that "we are seizing control of our own evolution".[26] These statements by leading figures in the field raise serious questions about their motivations and ethical perceptions. After the meeting the organizers made several policy recommendations to promote germ line gene therapy and to resist regulatory or legislative barriers to its exploration.

Concluding remarks

These issues should be discussed and decided with full public participation. Public interest organizations such as the Council for Responsible Genetics, patients and public health groups and concerned citizens should have a role in setting the agenda for policy forums, rather than just reacting to the formulations of scientists and bioethicists. Community and campus forums can air the issues in response to citizens' interests. Perhaps this would avoid the pattern in recent conferences where scientists involved in human genome projects and in gene transfer start off the program by explaining the science(and then leave), and the bioethicists remain to explain the ethical problems. Instead, interested citizens, students, faculty and patients' groups can decide what they need to know in order to make policy decisions. The "Science Shops" approach in the Netherlands and in Denmark might be useful, as would the "Community Research Network" being developed by the Loka Institute.[27]

Here are some criteria or guidelines to consider for this important process of public decision making regarding human genetic intervention:

Disclose fully any potential conflicts of interest.

Examine and challenge assumptions about progress and research freedom.

Refrain from simplistic genetic causality and misconceptions that specific genes will be discovered for complex genetic traits.

Avoid the loose language and exaggerations of genetic reductionism and the misleading claims of biohype.

Seek moral, scientific, medical and social policy alternatives and consider diverse views within the research community, the public health field, and public interest and consumer groups.

Set research priorities to meet public health needs rather than commercial goals.

Develop increased public literacy among scientists and a stronger sense of social responsibility by exposing them to the writing and thinking of others in the history, ethics, politics and sociology of the life sciences.

Do it sooner rather than defer it until it is too late.

Notes

1. I am completing a book on the history of social responsibility in science which will contain detailed accounts of these efforts.
2. Tiselius, 1961, pp. 14–15. See also Wiskari, 1961 and Kekwick,Pedersen, 1974, p. 416.
3. Several of the historical accounts that follow have been included in Weiner, 1994.
4. *New York Times*, 1962.
5. *New York Times*, 1963.
6. Hollaender, 1966.
7. Zinder, 1966.
8. Nirenberg, 1967.
9. Kass, 1967. Kass was responding to Lederberg, 1967a. See also Lederberg, 1967b.
10. Reinhold, 1969.
11. Shapiro, Eron, and Beckwith, 1969.
12. Beckwith, 1970.
13. Beckwith, 1993.
14. Pontecorvo, 1971, pp. 119–120.
15. Fox and Littlefield, 1971.
16. Anderson, 1972, pp. 109–110.
17. United States Senate, 1968.
18. Kass, 1970. See also, Krimsky, 1982, pp. 33–36.
19. Asilomar, 1975. Audiotape of the International Conference on Recombinant DNA Molecules (Asilomar Conference), February 24, 1975. Recombinant DNA History Collection, MIT Institute Archives and Special Collections.
20. Gustafsson, Rydén, Tibell, Wallensteen, 1984.
21. Gustafsson and Tibell, 1989, p. 72. See Rydén, 1990 for a full discussion of the code and the response to it.
22. Annas, 1989, p. 21.
23. Interview, 1984.
24. Kass, 1997, especially pp. 24–26, provides a perceptive critique of the response of the field of bioethics to human cloning. The same criticism is applicable to the response of many bioethicists to human germ line interventions.
25. Wade, 1998.
26. Quotations are from the proceedings as published on the website.
27. Information on these approaches can be found on the Loka Institute website, http://www.loka.org.

Bibliography

Anderson, F., 1972. "Genetic therapy." In: Hamilton, M. (ed.). *The New Genetics and the Future of Man*. Eerdmans: Grand Rapids, MI, pp.109–124.

Annas, G. J., 1989. "Who's afraid of the human genome?" *Hastings Center Report*, July/August, p. 21.

Beckwith, J. R., 1970. "Gene expression in bacteria and some concerns about the misuse of science." *Bacteriological Reviews* 34, 3, pp. 222–227.

Beckwith, J., 1993. "A historical view of social responsibility in genetics." *BioScience* 43, 5, pp. 327–333.

Fox, M., Littlefield, J., 1971. "Reservations concerning gene therapy." Editorial. *Science* 173, p. 195.

Gustafsson, B., Rydén, L., Tibell, G., Wallensteen, P., 1984. "The Uppsala code of ethics for scientists." *Journal of Peace Research* 21, 4, pp. 311–316.

Gustafsson, B., and Tibell, G., 1989. "Critics of science and research ethics in Sweden." *Philosophy and Social Action* 15, 3–4, pp. 60–74.

Hollaender, A., 1966. "Rockefeller University meeting on genetic intervention in humans, 1966." *Alexander Hollaender Papers*. American Philosophical Society Library: Philadelphia.

Kass, L. R, 1967. "Genetic tampering." Letter to the editor. *Washington Post*, November 3.

Kass, L., 1970. Letter to Paul Berg, October 30, 1970. Recombinant DNA History Collection, Massachusetts Institute of Technology Archives and Special Collections. Reproduced in: Krimsky, 1982, pp. 33–36.

Kass, L., 1997. "The wisdom of repugnance." *New Republic*, June 2, pp. 17–26.

Kekwick, R. A., Pedersen, K.O., 1974. "Arne Tiselius 1902–1971." *Biographical Memoirs of Fellows of the Royal Society* 20, pp. 401–428.

Krimsky, S., 1982. *Genetic Alchemy: The Social History of the Recombinant DNA Controversy*. MIT: Cambridge, MA.

Lederberg, J., 1967a. "Unpredictable variety still rules human reproduction." *Washington Post*, September 30.

Lederberg, J., 1967b. "Genetic intervention is a way of improving our species." *Washington Post*, November 4.

New York Times, 1962. "The code of life." Editorial, January 28.

New York Times, 1963. "Probing heredity's secrets." Editorial, September 12.

Nirenberg, M., 1967. "Will society be prepared?" Editorial, *Science*, August 11, p. 633.

Pontecorvo, G., 1971. In: Fuller, W. (ed.). *The Biological Revolution: Social Good or Social Evil?* Anchor, Doubleday: New York, pp. 119–120.

Reinhold, R., 1969. "Scientists isolate a gene; step in hereditary control." *New York Times*, November 23, p. 1.

Rydén, L., 1990 (ed.). Etik för forskare: En antologi med utgångspunkt i arbetet med Uppsalakodexen. UHÄ FoU: Stockholm.

Shapiro, J., Eron, L., Beckwith, J., 1969. Letter to the editor. *Nature* 224, December 27, p. 1337.

Tiselius, A., 1962. "Discours solonnel." *Les prix Nobel en 1961*. Norstedt & Söner: Stockholm, pp. 14–15.

United States Senate, 1968. Hearings before the Subcommittee on Government Research of the Committee on Government Operations, U.S. Senate, 90th Congress, 2nd Session, on S.J. Res. 145, a joint resolution for the establishment of the National Commission on Health, Science & Society, March 7, 8, 21, 22, 27, 28 and April 2, 1968, p. 5.

Wade, N., 1998. "Human cells revert to embryo state, scientists assert." *New York Times*, November 12, pp. 1, 24.

Weiner, C., 1994. "Anticipating the consequences of genetic engineering: past, present, and future." In: Cranor, C., (ed.). *Are Genes Us? The Social Consequences of the New Genetics*. Rutgers: New Brunswick, NJ, pp. 31–51.

Wiskari, N., 1961. "Scientists urged to be forthright: Nobel unit head bids them speak out to politicians." *New York Times*, December 17.

Zinder, N., 1966. "Summary of a meeting held on October 1, 1966 at the Rockefeller University." *Recombinant DNA History Collection*, MIT Institute Archives, pp. 1–7.

Conceptual Issues and Their Etical Implications

SIGRID GRAUMANN

Some Conceptual Questions about Somatic Gene Therapy and their Relevance for an Ethical Evaluation

Right from the beginning the development of molecular biology has been accompanied by the idea of making man himself the object of molecular genetic research:

> The highest level of application of molecular biology would be the direct control of nucleotid sequences in human chromosoms associated with the possibility to identify, select and integrate the desired genes which appear in an existing population in great variety.[1]

Ever since the genetic manipulation of mammal cells has been made possible, researchers have discussed a medical application of gene transfer technology on human beings. In the beginning public opinions tended to be rather sceptical towards plans concerning the genetic manipulation of human cells. "Considering that nuclear energy threatens global catastrophe and that many other technological advances visibly damage the quality of life, who would wish to have scientists tampering with man's inner nature."[2]

In addition to its success, modern technology brought about a general insecurity as the part of the public concerning its destructive potential. However, a still more relevant factor was that critics have placed genetic therapy in a historical context of fantasies about the improvement of man triggered by old as well as new eugenics. That is why a clear cut division between somatic gene therapy and germ line therapy has been decisive for the development of a concept of genetic therapy which has become publicly legitimised. Somatic gene therapy means that not all the cells of an organism are the target of genetic manipulation, but merely the pathologically relevant cells of specific tissue or organs. This means that genetic manipulations will not be passed on to descendants and that there is therefore no reason to fear modern technologies might serve as a basis for a genetic improvement of mankind. The concept of germ line therapy, however, is related to the idea of a direct manipulation of the germ cells of an organism, or all cells and this implies those germ cells as well which carry technically caused genetic manipulations and will thus be passed on to following generations. "The two issues—somatic cell gene therapy and germ line therapy—had to be distinguished and separated for purposes of debate and public policy considerations."[3]

In addition to this, a clear therapeutic orientation played a significant role in legitimizing gene therapy. Friedmann, who played an important role in the development of this concept, said: "The term gene therapy was adopted to distinguish itself from the ominous, germ-line perceptions of the term human genetic engineering."[4] Subsequently, it has been stated in general that there are no considerable objections to somatic gene therapy with a clear therapeutic aim. The following ethical discussion is restricted to the conditions of the clinical practice of somatic gene therapy[5]—and that means it is mainly concerned with the assessment of chances and risks.

This concept of somatic gene therapy which had shed its historical burden, became for many euphoric critics the object of hopes and promises. It appeared able to offer therapies against genetically caused diseases, which formerly could only be imperfectly treated if at all, by now being able to target their genetic basis. A revolution of traditional medicine was proclaimed. I would, however, argue, that the primary question would have to be, whether there is a possibility after all to realise this concept in accordance with its formulated goals. This is the first point where in my opinion basic doubts are justified.

Generally, risks have to be taken into consideration. The general rule for the legitimization of a therapy or a clinical trial demands, that the anticipated benefits for the involved patients have to overrule the risks. The presumption here is that the benefits as well as the risks can be determined. This is the second point where in my opinion basic doubts are justified.

The following reflection concerning the concept of somatic gene therapy will clarify these doubts.

Development and modification of the concept of somatic gene therapy

The original ideal concept of genetic therapy is to treat patients suffering from monogenetically caused hereditary diseases with a transfer of intact gene sequences on to the pathogenetically relevant cells and to thereby provide them with a causal, specific treatment that has relatively few side effects. "One approach of gene therapy would involve specific removal from the genome of a mutant gene sequence and its replacement with a normal functional gene."[6] In order to realise this idea it would have to be possible to implant the intact gene at exactly the same place as the defect gene in the genome of the target cell. This would theoretically guarantee that the therapeutic gene is exprimated correctly by its according regulating environment. This means, that the gene product would have to be produced in the right cell, at the right moment in the right amount and in the right relation to other proteins. This, however, is exactly what cannot be achieved with the transfer systems which are currently available for somatic therapy. The transfer gene integrates somewhere in the genome or is exprimated extrachromosomally. Therefore the effects of the gene transfer cannot be predicted with certainty.

This is the reason why in the first clinical tests only those diseases could be treated which were caused by the defect of a gene which did not necessarily have to be specifically regulated in order to achieve a therapeutic effect. Anderson, who performed the first clinical test in the field of gene therapy in 1990, said: "Early attempts in gene therapy will almost certainly be done with genes for enzymes that have a simple, 'always on' type of regulation."[7] Among these simple diseases are e.g. ADA-deficiency, cystic fibrosis and hypercholesterolaemia, which became the objects of the first clinical trials in the field of gene therapy of hereditary diseases.

Today, the great majority of clinical minutes is not about the treatment of monogenic hereditary diseases as was expected at first, but about the treatment of cancer and other acquired diseases which are regulated by environmental factors and a greater number of genes. All of the diverse strategies made use of in clinical tests in the field of gene therapy concerning the treatment of cancer aim at a reduction of the tumour mass and not at all at the genetic defects which may cause cancer. In this respect they do not differ in principle from conventional approaches in cancer treatment like the surgical removal of tumours, chemotherapy and radiation treatment. These concepts are not at all in accordance with the original idea of a specific gene correction or with the intention to triumph over diseases by targeting their genetic roots.

Gene therapy in the context of bio-medical research

The "Panel to Assess the NIH Investment in Research on Gene Therapy" in the United States asserted in its report published in December 1995 that up to now not a single successful clinical test has been made. Nevertheless somatic gene therapy is still associated with a special quality of medical progress:

> Somatic gene therapy is a logical and natural progression in the application of fundamental biomedical science to medicine and offers extraordinary potential, in the long-term, for the management and correction of human disease, including inherited and acquired disorders, cancer, and AIDS.[8]

The belief in future success, which is formulated here despite the fact that basic technical problems remain unresolved, can hardly be understood on a basis of established facts, but rather has to be regarded in a context of a Baconian optimism concerning progress: Scientific medicine, that is bio-medicine, is, according to Bacon's ideal associated with the notion of reliability, efficiency and success. The self-image of scientific medicine is based on the belief that it will be able to provide the most appropriate method in the fight against man's morbidity and mortality through participation in modern science research programs. Scientific methods are associated with the notion of exact and realistic documentation of phenomena, especially as long as the following three methodological rules are obeyed:

1. The abstraction of the singular concrete case to the ideal circumstances, the reduction of the research object to its methodologically relevant features.
2. The carrying out of controlled experiments. Only a few specific features of the object are observed and measured under controlled circumstances.
3. The formalised generalisation.

The goal of experimental scientific work is to gain control of the object of research. The methodological directive in doing so is to split the object into smaller and smaller empirically definable units in order to reconstruct it according to its smallest analysed units. The starting point for the development of the research program in the field of scientific medicine was made by the experimental physiologist Bernard (1813–1877).

> Consequently, the physiologist and the physician, as well as the physicist and the chemist who find themselves confronted with a complex question have to split up the whole of the problem again and again into simpler and better defined aspects.[9]

In the course of progress, the research program went from a macro to a micro level, from the level of organs to that of tissues, to the cells and finally to the DNA. Human genetics and especially gene therapy thus represent the temporary final point within the logic of the research program of scientific medicine, which Bernard had formulated already in the 19th century.

Questions concerning risks and methodical reductionism

A practical and theoretical simplification of reality is a prerequisite for the control of biological phenomena. The scientific formation of cognition assumes a reduction of complexity and always leads to reductionist interpretations in so far as certain aspects which are considered to be of major importance are placed in the centre and others become marginalised. This way of finding a way to deal with the phenomena is achieved by paying the price of a loss of reality which opens space for cognitive insights at the same time as it narrows down perspectives. A widening of cognition can be asserted in terms of the success of modern science. The narrowing of cognition caused by a loss of insight due to a selective perspective which is part of the approach has been widely criticised. On the one hand criticism was directed against incalculable risks brought about by modern science and technology, while on the other hand it was directed against the incapability to describe complex phenomena adequately.[10]

Gene therapy and the central genetic dogma

The development of somatic gene therapy as well as the major part of the entire genetic research is guided by three theoretical presumptions which may be called the central genetic dogma according to Francis Crick:

The first theoretical presumption is that the genotype represents a sophisticated chemical program, which controls all physiological processes including the development of an organism. The phenotype consequently represents the realisation of the genetic program.

The second theoretical presumption can be described as the one-dimensionality of genes. The sequence hypothesis, which Francis Crick formulated in 1957, assumes "that the peculiarity of a piece of nucleic acid is expressed only by the base sequence and that this sequence is a simple code for the amino acid of a specific protein."[11]

The third theoretical presumption is that the relationship between genotype and phenotype is a hierarchical one. This means that the flow of direction of information is from the DNA via the RNA to the protein.

Thus it is assumed that a mutation which can be found in a genome corresponds to a precisely relatable effect within the organism and that a technically caused genetic change would have to lead to a precisely predictable effect. If then a gene is transferred to certain cells of the body in the course of a somatic gene therapy treatment, the achievement of a precisely predictable therapeutic effect would have to be possible—assuming that the basic methodical problems are solvable. A prerequisite for such a success, however, is that the theoretical presumptions are correct.

Dispute about paradigms in the field of genetics

The central genetic dogma can be regarded in accordance with Thomas Kuhn as part of the leading paradigm of genetic research, which has to be unquestioningly accepted by the scientific community and on the basis of which ordinary scientific puzzle solving is carried out. According to Kuhn scientific progress proceeds in successive stages. The prescientific stage, which is characteristic of the relatively uncoordinated research of individual scientists is followed by an ordinary scientific stage in which a research-guiding paradigm is developed. A paradigm consists of general theoretical assumptions and rules as well as of techniques necessary for their application, which are accepted by the scientific community for a specific field of science. Ordinary research is practised by those scientists who operate within a paradigm. They have to adopt an uncritical attitude towards the paradigm. Their task is to do ordinary research within the realm of accepted means given by the paradigm—which would in this case be the molecular genetic resort of methods. The Human Genome Project would represent a striking example of ordinary scientific puzzle solving.

At the ordinary scientific stage empirical data repeatedly appear which question the dominant paradigm. However, this alone does not suffice to render the dominant paradigm obsolete. It is only when such anomalies accumulate and alternative paradigms become formulated that ordinary research finds itself in a crisis, which could lead to a revolutionary stage and to the establishment of a new paradigm.[12]

Voices have been raised which consider genetic research to be in such a stage of crisis. I do not want to determine at this moment whether they are right in proclaiming that the genetic paradigm has reached its end.[13] On the contrary, I rather doubt that because there are no methodological alternatives to the leading paradigm, only theoretical ones. However, I would like to present some empirical arguments in favour of this thesis and to make use of them for my own purposes:

Empirical arguments against the validity of the central genetic dogma

According to the central genetic dogma all regulation processes of organisms and cells which means the regulation of the development of organisms and the regulation of metabolic processes must be determined by the genes. But this is inconsistent with the popular understanding of metabolic processes as control circuit systems.[14] Accordingly regulative processes are envisioned as an interaction of gene, gene product and environment. E.g., the blood insulin concentration has to vary according to the blood sugar concentration. This means that the insulin-gene has to respond somehow to the environmental information 'sugar-concentration'. This contradicts the genetic dogma.

The genetic dogma contains the idea that ontogenesis proceeds in programatically regulated, additive and hierarchically structured sequences of developmental steps. However, the complicated and in this case necessary spatial and temporal co-ordination of the individual steps of development and differentiation cannot be explained satisfactorily in this way.[15]

More recent state of knowledge in genetics shows that the regulation of gene expression is not restricted to the level of the DNA. There are regulation mechanisms which are put up in front of the level of the DNA like DNA-imprinting.[16] And there are regulation mechanisms which succeed the transcription on the level of the RNA like m-RNA-splicing and m-RNA-editing.[17] We know DNA-sequences which deliver different gene products by these mechanisms. This means that there are regulation processes which cause alterations of the gene products beyond the DNA and therefore they are unlikely determined by the DNA alone.

In addition, we know physiological functions in the organisms which can be reached by different genetic path ways.[18] Such examples show that the DNA is not simply active but rather reactive to the necessities of life processes.

In order to describe complex phenomena like metabolic processes, development and gene expression, researchers today often fall back on explanation-models based on system theories:

One relatively simple alternative model concerning the regulation of metabolic processes and ontogenesis is derived from cybernetic control circuit models. A regulative network which is comprised of individual regulative units could be completed by other regulative elements on the level of DNA, RNA or gene product. By this means, cascade control units and feed back loops could be integrated as well.[19]

In the meantime more far reaching alternatives based on complex system theories gained acceptance in the formulation of biological theory. These alternative approaches consider interactive epigenetic networks to be the key to an understanding of physiological and ontogenetical regulative processes instead of the genom itself. Ontogenesis is in this case understood as a historical and not as a programmatic process, which is controlled by genetic and epigenetic interactions at all levels of organisation. Thus the phenotype represents the result of interactions between multiple factors, of which genes only represent one category.[20]

I do not agree with the opinion, that these explanation-models based on complex system theories can compensate for the reductionist deficits characteristic of the empirical-analytical methods of modern science. However, due to their adoption of a new perspective, that is, due to an analysis of the whole instead of particular elements only, these models help to broaden the understanding of biological phenomena.

Can gene therapy be considered a sensible goal of modern medicine?

If these alternative models of biological regulative processes prove to be of a higher validity and are thereby closer to empirical reality than the old genetic paradigm which has become doubtful, this would imply that the effects a natural genetic change or a technical genetic manipulation have on the phenotype are not exactly predictable. I do not argue that it is impossible to achieve certain desired effects, but simply that such effects cannot be predicted on a secure basis. Gene therapy tests would then be trial and error tests with a relatively undefined result and not as it was hoped calculated corrections of genetic deficiencies. It may be the case, that somatic gene therapy can enrich modern medicine with some new methods of treatment, but it can never, as has often been assumed bring about a revolution of scientific medicine. In addition to this, not only are the positive effects not exactly predictable; neither can the risks of gene therapy be calculated satisfactorily.

Implications for the ethical discussion

This perception is of particular relevance for the ethical evaluation of somatic gene therapy. On the one hand, those ethical arguments in favour of the novelty of therapeutically actions connected with somatic gene therapy lose their validity. The utility of gene transfer techniques in clinical practice will not be so huge and revolutionary as it has been assumed so far. In this respect, a policy of research which concentrates on the development of somatic gene therapy appears to be highly questionable, especially taking into consideration the limited nature of resources. In particular the development of alternative and perhaps more successful therapeutic approaches may become neglected thereby.

On the other hand, those ethical arguments objecting to somatic gene therapy by assuming that gene therapy cannot be restricted to therapeutic purposes for individual patients loose their validity as well. If the above mentioned thesis is true, it will be impossible to achieve exactly calculated effects in humans. This means that both hopes and fears about total genetic control by gene therapy or genetic enhancement are extremely unrealistic.

It follows that, we should concentrate on the assessment of chances and risks of somatic gene therapy by taking into account the uncertainty of the achievable goals and by taking the biological risks of gene transfer in humans more seriously.

Because of the methodological problems and the uncertainty of the theoretical basis of gene therapy we cannot state today that the anticipated benefits for the involved patients outweigh the risks. This means that up to now the general rule for the legitimisation of therapies or clinical trials cannot be fulfilled. We do not know what exactly future scientific progress may bring. We can assume that it will not provide us with a revolution in medicine by overcoming genetic diseases. We can rather hope that it will offer some additional symptomatic but nevertheless useful therapeutic options. And we know that it is of decisive importance to assess the risks of gene transfer carefully before introducing somatic gene therapy into (experimental) clinical practice.

Notes

1. Lederberg, 1962.
2. Davis, 1970.
3. Fletcher, 1990.
4. Friedmann, 1990.
5. Rehmann-Sutter, Müller 1995, p. 20.
6. Friedmann, 1989.
7. Anderson, 1984.
8. NIH-Report 12/95.
9. Bernard, 1991, p. 106.
10. Bonss, Hohlfeld, Kollek, 1992.
11. Crick, 1990, p. 149.
12. Kuhn, 1962.
13. Strohman, 1997.
14. Jacob, Monod, 1961.
15. Stent, 1985.
16. Lalande, 1997.
17. Chabot, 1996; Navaratnam et al., 1995.
18. Jiang et al., 1993; Tautz, 1992; Wagner, 1996.
19. Crow, Dove, 1990.
20. Strohman, 1994, 1997; Wolf, 1995, 1998.

Bibliography

Anderson, W. F., 1984. "Prospects for human gene therapy." *Science* 226, pp. 401–409.

Anderson, W. F., 1990. "The beginning." *Human Gene Therapy* 1, pp. 371–372.

Bacon, F., 1962. *Das neue Organon*. Academie-Verlag: Berlin.

Bernard, C., 1991. *Einführung in das Studium der experimentellen Medizin* (Paris 1865). Barth: Leipzig.

Böhme, G., 1977. "Die kognitive Ausdifferenzierung der Naturwissenschaft. Newtons mathematische Naturphilosophie." In: Böhme, G., van den Daele, W., Krohn, W. (eds.). *Experimentelle Philosophie. Ursprünge autonomer Wissenschaftentwicklung*. Suhrkamp: Frankfurt, p. 237–263.

Bonss, W., Hohlfeld, R., Kollek, R., 1992. "Risiko und Kontext. Zum Umgang mit den Risiken der Gentechnologie." In: Bechmann, G., Rammert, W. (eds.). *Technik und Gesellschaft.* Jahrbuch 6, Frankfurt a. M., p.141–174.

Bonss, W., Hohlfeld, R., Kollek, R., 1994. "Vorüberlegungen zu einem kontextualistischen Modell der Wissenschaftsentwicklung." *Deutsche Zeitschrift für Philosophie* 42, 3, pp. 439–454.

Chabot, B., 1996. "Directing alternative splicing: Cast and scenarios." *Trends in Genetics* 12, 11, pp. 472–478.

Crick, F., 1988. *What Mad Pursuit: a Personal View of Scientific Discovery.* Basic Books: New York.

Crick, F., 1990 *Ein irres Unternehmen. Die Doppelhelix und das Abenteuer Molekularbiologie.* Piper: München.

Crow, J. F., Dove, W. F., 1990. "Genes and development: Molecular and logical themes." *Genetics* 126, pp. 479–486.

Davis, B. D., 1970. "Prospects for genetic intervention in man." *Science* 170, pp. 1279–1283.

Fletcher, J. C., 1990. "Evolution of ethical debate about human gene therapy." *Human Gene Therapy* 1, pp. 55–68.

Friedmann, T., 1989. "Progress toward human gene therapy." *Science* 244, pp. 1275–1281.

Friedmann, T., 1990. "The Evolving Concept of Gene Therapy." *Human Gene Therapy* 1: pp. 175–181.

Gilbert, W., 1991. "Towards a Paradigm Shift in Biology." *Nature* 349, p. 99.

Hess, B., Mikhailov, A., 1994. "Self-organizing in living cells." *Science* 264, pp. 223–224.

Jacob F., Monod, J., 1961. "Genetic regulatory mechanisms in the synthesis of proteins." *Journal of Molecular Biology* 3, pp. 318–356.

Jiang, C., Finkbeiner, W. E., Widdicombe, J. H., McCray, P. B., Miller, S. S., 1993. "Altered fluid transport across airway epithelium in cystic fibrosis." *Science* 262, pp. 424–427.

Kollek, R., 1997. "Risikokonzepte: Strategien zum Umgang mit Unsicherheit in der Gentechnik." In: Elstner, M. (Hrsg.). *Gentechnik, Ethik und Gesellschaft.* Springer: Berlin, Heidelberg, pp. 123–140.

Krohn, G., Küppers, G. (Hrsg.). 1992. *Emergenz: die Entstehung von Ordnung, Organisation und Bedeutung.* Suhrkamp: Frankfurt a.M.

Kuhn, T. S., 1962. *The structure of scientific revolution.* University of Chicago Press: Chicago.

Lalande, M., 1997. "Parental imprinting and human disease." *Annual Review Genetics* 31, pp. 173–195.

Lederberg, J., 1962. "Biological Future of Man." In: Jungk, R., Mundt, H.J. (eds.). *Das umstrittene Experiment: Der Mensch.* Dokumentation des Ciba-Symposiums 1962. (*Man and His Future.* Campus Verlag: Frankfurt a. M., München, 1988.)

Leff, S. E., Evans, R. M., Rosenfeld, M. G., 1987. "Splice commitment dictates neuron-specific alternative RNA-processing in calcitonin/CGRP gene expression." *Cell* 48, pp. 517–524.

Louis, D. N., Gusella, J. F., 1995. "A tiger behind many doors: Multiple genetic pathways to malignant glioma." *Trends in Genetics*10, 11, pp. 412–415.

Madhani, H. D., Guthrie, C., 1994. "Dynamic RNA-RNA interactions in the spliceosome." *Annual Review Genetics* 28, pp. 1–26.

Monk, M., 1995. "Epigenetic programming of differential gene expression in development and evolution." *Developmental Genetics* 17, 3, pp. 188–197.

Müller, R., 1995. "Transcriptional regulation during the mammalian cell cycle." *Trends in Genetics* 11, 5, pp. 173–178.

Müller, S., Simon, J. W., Vesting, J. W. (eds.). *Interdisciplinary approaches to gene therapy.* Springer: Berlin, Heidelberg, New York.

Navaratnam, N., Bhattacharya, S., Fujino, T., Patel, D., Jarmuz, A. L., Scott, J., 1995. "Evolutionary origins of apoB mRNA editing: Catalysis by a cytidine deaminase that has acquired a novel RNA-binding motif at its active site." *Cell* 81, 2, pp. 187–195.

Nijhout, H. F., 1990. "Metaphors and the role of genes in development." *BioEssays* 12, 9, pp. 441–446.

Nilsen, R. W., 1994. "RNA-RNA interactions in the spliceosome: Unraveling the ties that bind." *Cell* 78, pp. 1–4.

Orkin, S. H., Motulsky, A. D., 1995. Report and recommendations of the Panel to Assess the NIH Investment in Research on Gene Therapy. NIH: Bethesda.

Rehmann-Sutter, C., Müller, H. (eds.), 1995. *Ethik und Gentherapie. Zum praktischen Diskurs um die molekulare Medizin.* Francke: Tübingen.

Sharp, P. A., 1994. "Split genes and RNA splicing." Nobel lecture. *Cell* 77, pp. 805–815.

Stent, G. S., 1985. "Thinking in one dimension: the impact of molecular biology on development." *Cell* 40, pp. 1–2.

Strohman, R., 1994. "Epigenesis: the missing beat in biotechnology." *Biotechnology* 12, pp. 156–164.

Strohman, R. C., 1997. "The coming Kuhnian revolution in biology. Epigenesis and complexity." *Nature Biotechnology* 15, pp. 194–200.

Tautz, D., 1992. "Redundancies, development and the flow of information." *Bio Essays* 14, 4, pp. 263–266.

Wagner, A., 1996. "Genetic redundancy caused by gene duplications and its evolution in networks of transcriptional regulators." *Biological Cybernetics* 74, pp. 557–567.

Wolf, U., 1995. "The genetic contrubution to the phenotype." *Human Genetics* 95, pp. 127–148.

Wolf, U., 1998. "Identical mutations and phenotypic variation." *Human Genetics*100, pp. 305–321.

Wolff, J. A., Lederberg, J., 1994. "An early history of gene transfer and therapy." *Human Gene Therapy* 5, p. 469–480.

Wu, J. Y., Maniatis, T., 1993. "Specific interactions between proteins implicated in splice site selection and regulated alternative splicing." *Cell* 75, pp. 1061–1070.

KAREN LEBACQZ

The Ambiguities of 'Therapy' and their Implications for the Place of Women and the Disabled in a Gene-Focused Society

Virgil's story[1]

Virgil was born on a small farm in the early 1940s. Even as a small child, his vision was not good, but after a devastating illness at around age six, both his retinas were severely damaged. He developed thick cataracts and was sent to a school for the blind. There he learned to read Braille and became adept at getting around with a cane. When he graduated, he trained in massage and got a job as a massage therapist. In 1991, somewhat by chance, he re-encountered a woman he had met some 20 years before; they began to spend time together, and eventually became engaged. Amy refused to believe that Virgil's eyes were permanently blinded, and she finally found a surgeon willing to remove the cataracts. With the removal of the cataracts, in spite of the significant retinal damage that Virgil had sustained as a small child, he could indeed see colors and shapes. His sight appeared to be at least partially restored.

In the Bible (e.g., Mark 8:22–25), this image of the blind being given the gift of sight and suddenly seeing is used as a symbol of the joy of transformation. So we would expect that Virgil and those who loved him would leap for joy at his restored sight. And so they did—at first.

However, the story is not so simple. Virgil could indeed see colors and shapes, but he had no idea what those colors and shapes *were*—what they *meant*. He could recognize letters (which he had previously learned to recognize by feel), but he was unable to see a block of letters together and see a *word* made of those letters. Thus, he could distinguish the letters "C," "A," and "T" but could not see them together as the word "CAT." The tactile world in which Virgil had lived for so long is a *sequential* world composed of feeling one thing after another. The visual world is *simultaneous*. Virgil was not prepared for this, and had no basis in experience for understanding it. Nor could he put together the multiple visual inputs that would allow him to tell his cat from his dog (both were the same color!); he could distinguish them only if he closed his eyes and *felt* the animals in the way that had been his custom for more than 40 years. Using sight alone, Virgil could distinguish objects, but he had no sense of how close or distant they were and sometimes jumped back to protect himself from things that in fact were very far away.

In other words, Virgil received the 'gift' of sight, but not the gift of perception or meaningful sight. Seeing is not a simple matter of having images implant on our retinas. We do not simply 'see.' We *learn* to see. We learn to take the multitude of visual inputs and distinguish meaningful patterns out of them. Virgil had 40 years of being blind. He had never learned to see.

Worse yet, it is not clear that he *could* learn to see at this late date. As a sighted child grows, experiences are catalogued and the brain adapts and develops in order to process what our eyes take in. Indeed, in a seeing person, roughly half of the cerebral cortex is taken up by sight. Having not had sight before, it is possible that regions of the Virgil's cerebral cortex that normally develop to enable visual perception had been adapted instead to tactile or auditory reception. (Like many blind people, Virgil appeared to have acute hearing.) These regions might then not be available for developing meaningful sight.

In short, Virgil had now been given a physical capacity—the ability to receive images on the retina—for which he had no experiential substrate and for which additional physical capacities (cortical activity) that would have enabled him to *use* his new-found sight were likely missing.[2] Virgil 'saw,' but not in ways that were meaningful or helpful to him, and it was not clear that he could develop such meaningful or helpful ways. He was still most comfortable using his tactile sense to 'know' things. It is not clear that being given sight actually expanded Virgil's range of capacities, or ever would.

Even worse, though, Virgil was now *treated* as a non-blind person. He was expected to have and use sight in ways that were meaningful, even though he could not in fact do so. At the end of his poignant treatise on Virgil, Oliver Sacks remarks that Virgil "found himself between two worlds, at home in neither—a torment from which no escape seemed possible."[3]

Virgil's experience of being between two worlds, and not being able to adapt to a seeing world, is not unusual among those who have been long blind and then given the 'gift' of sight. Although some patients do manage to adapt to a seeing world, more commonly they find themselves precisely in the 'in between' state that Virgil experienced. Sacks notes that another patient "was first delighted with seeing, but soon encountered intolerable stresses and difficulties, found the 'gift' transformed to a curse, became deeply depressed, and soon after died."[4]

Ironically, release from this torment did finally come for Virgil when he contracted another disease that nearly killed him and left him once again functionally and legally blind, back in the world that Sacks calls the world of 'his own true being.'

Relevance to gene therapy

Virgil's condition was not genetic, the therapy used on Virgil was not gene therapy, and I do not propose that Virgil would have been a candidate for gene therapy. What, then, is the relevance of this story for a discussion of gene therapy? Virgil's story is relevant because it illustrates the deep chasm between the paradoxical and sometimes harsh realities of the real lived texture of our lives and the unambiguous hopes that we sometimes hold out for gene therapy. The reality is that therapy is often *ambiguous* while our hopes and myths about therapy are often *unambiguous.* We think of therapy as 'cure,' but in fact it is really an intervention—an intervention with mixed results. Later, I will show that treatment for some genetic conditions also shares in this quality of ambiguity, and that the ambiguities of therapy have significant implications for women and for those considered 'disabled' in society.[5]

In the popular mind, the image of gene therapy is something like this: We will locate a 'bad' gene and fix it (either in vivo or ex vivo) or replace it with a 'good' gene. Normal function will be restored, and the person will be 'cured' of what has ailed them. Our image of therapy is direct, clean, uncomplicated, straightforward. The model for therapy comes from acute illness: in cases of 'strep throat,' for example, we give penicillin which kills the streptococcus bacilli, the strep throat disappears, and the patient recovers to health.

At present, the reality of gene therapy is very far from this ideal image. In gene therapy, altered genetic material is inserted into a patient in hopes that it will find the right place to attach itself and that it will then be appropriately expressed, but there is no certainty that this will happen.[6] Part of the reason that most commentators are very hesitant to allow germ-line gene therapy is precisely because scientists have very little control over where the genes insert themselves and whether those genes will function correctly once inserted; the danger in germ-line therapy is that any mis-insertion or mal-function would be handed down through generations. But the popular hope—a hope shared by scientists—is that we will get to the point where we have more precision and more control, so that gene therapy will be a bit less like playing Russian Roulette (taking potentially deadly chances) and a bit more like giving penicillin to a patient suffering with strep throat. We assume that if we can get rid of the 'bad,' only 'good' ensues.

Virgil's case, however, illustrates that it is possible to remove a 'disease' or repair a body part (in Virgil's case, the eyes) without achieving the 'cure' or 'wholeness' or 'good' that we seek. Virgil's story illustrates the many deep complexities that have long plagued disability policy.[7] Is the restoration of sight or hearing a gift or a curse? What constitutes a 'disease' that should be 'fixed'? If we try to 'fix' deviations in adults, will we in fact end up demolishing something of the *substance* of who people are, making it difficult for them to find their own subjectivity? Should we allow those who have adapted well to the absence of a faculty such as sight or hearing to continue in their world of adaptation, or should we make every effort to 'restore' them and 'mainstream' them into dominant society? These questions are not new, but they are pertinent for helping us to 'see' (pardon the play on words!) both the possibilities and promises but also the perils and pitfalls of gene therapy. I will address only some of those pitfalls here: what constitutes disease or disability; the difference between loss of capacity and simple difference in capacity; the need for 'preparation' for therapy and change; the locus of disability—whether it is 'in' someone or 'out there' in society, socially constructed; the danger of 'geneticism'; and the implications for a feminist understanding of justice.

The definition of disability

Therapy implies that something is 'wrong' and needs to be 'fixed' or corrected. How do we know when we have a condition that is in need of being fixed or corrected? This is a hotly contested issue at present in disability studies.

In their thorough and generally excellent study, *The Ethics of Human Gene Therapy*, LeRoy Walters and Julie Gage Palmer suggest that a number of questions must be answered satisfactorily before experiments in gene therapy can proceed ethically. The very first of these questions is this: Is the disease *sufficiently serious* to merit treatment with an experimental technique?[8] All of the diseases of the first 100 protocols to be officially approved in the United States, they note, were for diseases that were either life-threatening or represented significant deviations from species-typical functioning. Thus, presumably, all 100 protocols fit the criterion of being *sufficiently serious* to merit such experimental intervention. Certainly one thinks here of children such as Ashanthi DeSilva, who was treated for Severe Combined Immune Deficiency syndrome (SCID)—a deadly disorder that threatened Ashanti's very life and for which she received gene therapy.[9]

While SCID is a "significant deviation from species-typical functioning," so is blindness or deafness. Some years ago, geneticist Bentley Glass took congenital blindness or deafness to be defects on which there would be shared consensus about seriousness; he assumed that therapy would be justified if it were available.[10] This is obviously the way Virgil's fiancee, Amy, also reasoned: since it is 'better' to have sight than to be blind, Virgil's sight should be restored if possible. But precisely here is the problem. When we say that a disease is sufficiently serious to merit intervention because it represents a "significant deviation from species-typical functioning," we have entered the world of value judgments about aberrations from the norm. Those aberrations may look very different from the "inside" than they do from the "outside."

Virgil's blindness was not simply a disease or disorder that Virgil 'had.' Virgil's blindness became part and parcel of *him.* He spent 40 years knowing the world as a blind person, and developing all the gifts that attend blindness, such as acute hearing and tactile discrimination. Virgil was a blind person who had adjusted extremely well to not having sight: he was educated, he held a steady job, he lived on his own, he planned to marry. Surely such accomplishments are normally taken as signs of successful living. While Virgil's blindness was an aberration from the norm, it did not prevent him from living a full life. As disability politics suggests, one might be in one's right mind and *not* want to get rid of aberrations from the norm.

This is the case where the Deaf are concerned.[11] The Deaf community is well organized and argues that deafness *per se* is not a disability but simply a difference, a deviation from species-typical functioning that can easily be accommodated by life in a community where Sign is the dominant language.[12] Most people who were born deaf will grow up in Deaf culture and see themselves *not* as people with a disability—the inability to hear—but rather as people who are primarily visual and belong to a distinct culture with its own social organization, language, history, and mores.[13] Indeed, they may consider those who can hear to be 'disabled' because we lack acute visual sense![14] The Deaf community rejects cochlear implants, for example.[15]

There is some indication that the 'Little People of America' who represent dwarfs and midgets (people of unusually short stature) take an analogous position, arguing that shortness is not a disability to be corrected but merely a difference to be accepted.[16] Ruth Ricker, past president of Little People of America, Inc. and a civil rights investigator for the U.S. Department of Education, anticipates that future technology will allow detection of many relatively common conditions in the first trimester of pregnancy.[17] The gene mutation for achondroplasia, identified in 1994, causes about half the instances of dwarfism and will probably be included in the DNA chip under development to be used in prenatal testing. The assumption in such testing would be that parents might choose not to have a child with dwarfism. But dwarfism, Ricker argues, is "on the cusp between disability and trait." Many dwarfs are short but have no medical or disabling complications. They are different but not disabled. Why should we assume that variations in height "represent brokenness and therefore need to be eliminated or otherwise fixed?" queries Ricker.

Hence, a "significant deviation from species-typical functioning" such as deafness or shortness is not *necessarily* a disability requiring or justifying intervention. From a sighted person's perspective, a blind person 'adapts' to the 'loss' of sight by developing acute hearing and excellent tactile sense. From a blind person's perspective, however, there is no 'loss' of sight, except perhaps for those who go blind later in life; rather, there is simply a different way of learning to perceive the world. Indeed, a blind person might say that a sighted person 'adapts' to an imperfection of hearing or of tactile sense by developing the ability to distinguish patterns through vision. Perspective counts! What is considered a 'disability' from the perspective of dominant culture is not necessarily a disability to those who deviate from the cultural norm. Not all difference is experienced as problematic. Freud's celebrated and controversial notion of 'penis-envy,' for example, is a theory based on an understanding that women's differences from men represent a problem, and that women 'envy' the male penis. But is this necessarily the case? Most feminists would today argue that it is not! Rather than focus on what women do *not* have, feminists focus on what women do have—a womb with the capacity to bear a child, and breasts with the capacity to suckle a child. Just as deaf people may experience deafness not as loss but as the presence of great visual acuity, and blind people may experience blindness not as loss but as the presence of great auditory acuity, so any difference may be looked at not as loss or problem but as *presence* and *capacity.*

Significant deviations from usual functioning are not, therefore, always understood as problematic from the perspective of those who carry such deviations, nor would they be seen as 'sufficiently serious' to justify therapy. This is the first ambiguity in trying to ascertain when gene therapy might be justified.

Absence, loss, presence, and capacity

Yet there clearly are circumstances in which people with differences *do* consider their conditions disabling and would gladly agree to 'therapy.' A recent documentary, drawn from the work of Oliver Sacks, followed the history of members of a select group of people who have Usher's syndrome.[18] Usher's syndrome is characterized by congenital deafness. People with Usher's syndrome therefore usually grow up using Sign as their primary language. Sign is an enormously *visual* language, in which the positioning of symbols in a particular place in the air carries part of the meaning of the symbol.[19] Hence, vision is crucial for those using Sign. Starting around age 16, people with Usher's syndrome who are already deaf also begin to go blind. They must switch from *visual* Sign language to a *tactile* version of Sign language. Regions of the cerebral cortex that have been taken over by vision must be readapted to tactile sensory input. (Virgil's story reminds us that adaptations from tactile to visual or the reverse may not be easy.)

Asked whether they would like to recover their vision, all of the people with Usher's syndrome quoted in the documentary said, 'yes.' Asked whether they would like to hear, all of them said, 'no.' The experience of those with Usher's syndrome suggests an additional possibility in thinking about warrants for gene therapy. Vision is something those with Usher's syndrome *had* and *lost.* Hearing is something they never experienced. They had a complete world without it. They had no sense of having 'lost' anything by not being able to hear. One can only lose what one has had. Those who have never had do not experience loss. So perhaps what is crucial is whether we *lose* something. When something has been lost and is restored, that restoration appears on the surface to represent a great gift. Certainly, this is the lesson that we might learn from those with Usher's syndrome, who have no desire to *hear*, as it is a capacity that they have never had and do not need in order to function well in their community, but do have a desire to *see,* as it is a capacity that they have had and lost, and that appears more central to well-being in their community.

Yet even this analysis would be too simplistic. There are circumstances where there has been no 'loss' per se, but where differences are experienced not simply as presence and capacity, as the disability rights movement might argue, but as problematic. For example, Tourette's syndrome is a disorder that may affect as many as one in a thousand people. Characterized by compulsive behaviors such as ritualized touching or jerking, and sometimes also by compulsive outbursts of speech, including swearing and other offensive statements, Tourette's syndrome is very uncomfortable for most people who have it, although many do find that they are able to work and can develop supportive and accepting communities around them.[20] Since Tourette's has a genetic base, it is possible that gene therapy will someday be available for Tourette's syndrome. What view would the Tourette's community take to the elimination of this disorder? Would gene therapy be chosen by those with Tourette's?

At first glance, we are tempted to say 'yes.' The Web sites associated with Tourette's suggest that many people with Tourette's would like to be 'cured' of their ritualistic and compulsive behaviors.[21] Rather than restoring a capacity that they have lost, they would like to *lose* what they have!

Yet again, this first glance is too simplistic. In his early book, *The Man Who Mistook His Wife for a Hat,* Oliver Sacks offers the case of "Witty Ticcy Ray." Ray was severely affected by Tourette's.[22] His tics and grimaces and verbal outbursts were constant during waking hours, and he had lost one job after another because of them. When treated with Haldol, Ray's movements subsided and he 'slowed down' to a more normal pace. But he felt that something was 'missing' in his life: although he was now able to work a steady job, he had lost the wild and creative surges that had made him a part-time musician of some extraordinary competence. Ray finally compromised by taking Haldol only some of the time and having two "selves"—what he called his 'Haldol' self of calmness during the work week, and his 'Ticcy' or Touretty self on weekends.

Ray's story, like Virgil's, illustrates that the 'self' that emerges following therapy may not be altogether comfortable. To give consent to an intervention that removes a core part of who one is and how one has adapted to the world is to consent to be a different person. Can one give informed consent to an intervention that in fact changes the very person who is giving the consent? These are troubling issues that must be faced if we are to undertake gene therapy. While many people with Tourette's would like to get rid of *some* of their symptoms, they might not in fact be happy if *all* of the symptoms of their current selves disappear. As Ray put it at one point, "Suppose you *could* take away the tics? What would be left? I consist of tics—there is nothing else."[23]

Moreover, since Tourette's syndrome has only recently been publicized, my prediction is that many people who have suffered with Tourette's would choose gene therapy if given that choice today. However, my prediction is also that within a few years, as information spreads about Tourette's and as those with the disease discover support communities through the Web and other sources, a movement will emerge to see Tourette's *not* as a disability in need of correction, but simply as a different way of being in the world that can be accepted and need not (for most people) make life unbearably difficult. Further, I suspect that if gene therapy were done for Tourette's syndrome, those who have formerly had the syndrome might find that they missed *themselves*, as they would no longer be the same person they were, and that (just as gaining sight when one has been blinded is not necessarily the 'gift' one anticipated) the adjustment to not having Tourette's might be far more difficult than anticipated. While many think that they would like to be freed of their compulsive behaviors, the actual state of being free of those behaviors might leave a sense of a void that needs to be filled, as it did for Ray.

The ambiguities of gene therapy thus include the possibility that things that we today think are 'obvious' candidates for therapy will not be in a few years when there is more political organization of different groups, just as Bentley Glass' assumption that deafness would be an 'obvious' candidate for therapy is undermined by the powerful existence of the Deaf community. Moreover, our consideration of the ambiguities of gene therapy must include the possibility that the 'self' we seek to cure becomes so different because of the therapy itself that we cannot say that we have indeed fixed anything, but may simply have changed it.

Preparing for therapy and 'allowing' miracles

The possibility that we have not *fixed* but only *changed* something leads to another concern. Sacks makes a telling comment in his analysis of Ray's case. While the effects of Haldol for Ray were 'miraculous,' he suggests, it was a miracle that had to be 'allowed.' The first time Ray was given Haldol, it not only slowed him down, it made him unable to function well. He was *too* slow; he could not react appropriately. For example, he got hit in the face by a revolving door because he could not move into it sufficiently quickly—a problem that he had never experienced while exhibiting Tourette's symptoms. He was not at all happy about his 'treatment.' Not until Ray had undergone some months of careful conversation and preparation for what it would mean to be non-Tourettish was he able to take Haldol without going into a physiological imbalance that moved him away from his tics but too far in the opposite direction. Preparation was needed so that the removal of the tics could be a gift rather than a curse—and even then, as we recall, the tics had to be restored part-time so that Ray did not lose the particular gifts that Tourette's brought into the musical portion of his life.

Sacks' reflection on 'allowing' miracles suggests two cautions as we encounter the possibilities of gene therapy for conditions such as Tourette's. First, even those characteristics that we consider unwanted, unhelpful, and useless may in fact become so much a part of ourselves that to get rid of them is to get rid of something of who we *are.*

In disability discussions, this problem is reflected in the language of 'being disabled' vs. 'having a disability.' While most people today prefer to speak of "having" a disability rather than "being" disabled, Susan Wendell notes that saying "I am disabled" may be important for taking personal ownership of one's situation, even though saying "I have a disability" helps to create solidarity with others whose disabilities are different.[24] Problems abound with either language: "I *am* disabled" tends to identify the person too much with the disability (e.g., we used to say "a mongoloid," as though Down syndrome completely identified the person), but "I *have* a disability" may not identify the depth and extent to which physical differences and their effects tend to create and modify personal identity. Precisely because differences do tend to create and modify identity, 'therapy' is not unambiguous. Most of us can readily see that the transition from being 'well' or 'normal' to being 'sick' or 'disabled' is an identity-changing and life-changing event: "Recognizing myself as disabled," writes Wendell, "certainly required that I change my self-identity and adopt a radically new way of thinking about myself."[25] But if "to become disabled is to enter a different world,"[26] so to have been disabled and become 'normal' is also to enter a different world, I would submit. Although temporarily non-disabled people[27] tend to think of our world as unambiguously good, that will not necessarily be the way that world appears to those who enter it after establishing an identity in a different world.

In any case, preparation may be necessary in order to enter that world. Sacks points out that in Mark's version of the story in which the blind man gained sight, the gain came in two stages. The healing was not complete and instantaneous, but took time and readjustment: first, the blind man saw people as trees walking, and only then came to see them as people. Biblical stories are full of this preparation for the jubilee moments. Preparation may come in the seeking, as in the woman who sought out Jesus and touched his cloak in order to heal herself. Preparation may come in forgiveness of sins, as when Jesus first said to the paralytic man, "your sins are forgiven," and only then "take up your bed and walk." This stage of preparation is crucial, and it cannot be ignored if we are to do gene therapy responsibly. One of the ambiguities of therapy is that it does not always appear therapeutic unless proper groundwork is laid.

The social construction of disability

Yet Sacks' claim about 'allowing' a miracle to happen also raises another, more problematic issue. In this early work, Sacks clearly does not take a 'disability rights' approach that would see Tourette's syndrome as a difference rather than a disability. Sacks claims that Ray had "no experience of any normal life."[28] Sacks here assumes that there is a 'normal' that can be defined and described, and that Tourette's does not fit that definition or description.[29] As Wendell notes, the power to define disability is not generally in the hands of those most affected by disability policies.[30] Yet some with Tourette's, like those who are Deaf or belong to Little People of America, might indeed say that they are not 'abnormal' but simply have a 'different' normality. After all, *all* of us carry aberrant genes. Many of us in academic professions are myopic—near-sighted. We do not consider ourselves *disabled* because we must wear glasses in order to drive a car, watch television, or see the faces of our students when we are lecturing. We accept wearing glasses or contact lenses as a normal part of our everyday routine. Just so does a person who is legally blind develop normal parts of an everyday routine that may not seem at all 'disabling' to that person. Just so does a person with compulsive behaviors develop routines that simply include those behaviors, however bizarre they may seem from the outside.

If having malfunctions makes us disabled, then almost *all* of us are disabled. If being able to adapt to those malfunctions makes us not disabled, then almost all of us are *not* disabled, even those who are generally labeled disabled by others. To say this is to raise a fundamental challenge as to whether disability is something that inheres *in* a person—a characteristic of the individual—or whether disability is something that society *constructs.* For example, Susan Wendell points out that in any society that continually increases the expectations of *pace* of life (what some of us call the 'rat race'), people are disabled not because they cannot *do* things, but because they cannot do them *fast enough* to meet expectations.[31] As one who herself has myalgic encephalomyelitis (called 'chronic fatigue syndrome' in the United States), Wendell notes that if members of her faculty were asked to carry an additional course per semester, her 'disability' would increase without any change in her physical status. In such subtle ways, she suggests, we create disability where there did not need to be any such: "the social response to and treatment of biological difference constructs disability from biological reality, determining both the nature and the severity of disability."[32] Similarly, differences such as shortness or inability to hear do not constitute disabilities *in themselves;* rather, these differences are *constructed as* disabilities by a society that insists on everything being done one way.[33] If education is entirely based on hearing, for example, deaf children will be disabled; but if education were based on both spoken *and* visual language, deaf children would not be disabled in the educational system.

In short, the language and territory of disability is itself contested ground,[34] and this contributes to the ambiguities of therapy. If disability does not exist, therapy is not needed. If disability is entirely socially constructed, then perhaps "therapy" should be geared not toward the individual and his or her genes but toward society: it is society and its reactions to difference that needs to be changed, not the individual. Only if there is a meaningful way in which to speak of disability and disease on an individual level does gene therapy become a useful concept. Whether there is such a meaningful way is itself contested ground today.

Implications for women and other 'disabled' people

What is the importance of all this from a feminist or woman's perspective? There was a time in Western history when women were indeed viewed as 'inferior' or 'inverted' males: men with their penises turned 'inside' to make a vagina and uterus.[35] Since maleness was the standard (as it still is in many ways in medicine), femaleness emerged as something deviant, wrong, inadequate. Would we have 'fixed' femaleness if we could? Would gene therapy have been appropriate in order to correct all those deficient males?

Would we fix women today? Of the 8000 abortions performed in one region of India a few years ago, all but three were of female fetuses. Would the parents of the 7997 'fix' the gender of their children if they could? Would they ask to have all those 'X' chromosomes turned into 'Y' chromosomes?

The danger for women as women, as well as the danger for women and other members of groups considered deviant or disabled by the dominant group, is that a *norm* or standard is set for what we *should* be. Those who do not fit the norm are then presumed to be inferior, inadequate, in need of therapy. As Roger Shinn puts it, "Lurking in all genetic theory and practice is the disturbing question of norms."[36] Put another way, lurking in all genetic theory and practice is the disturbing question of the 'normal.'

Shinn points out that 'normal' tends to mean 'usual.' Because it is 'usual' for us to have five fingers on each hand, for example, we assume that six fingers is 'abnormal.' Because heterosexuality is more 'usual' than homosexuality, we assume that heterosexuality is 'normal' and homosexuality 'abnormal.' I would add that, in medicine, 'normal' often means 'functional'—e.g., a 'normal' stomach is one that digests food, a 'normal' uterus is one that has the capacity to bear a child, and so on. Because it is 'usual' for people to see, or because this is the 'function' of eyes, we assume that not seeing is 'abnormal.' Normal does not mean without defect, then—it means fitting the usual pattern and/or being functional within some definition of acceptable functioning. Functions change over time and geography, and hence, definitions of the 'normal' will also change. For instance, a 'normal' uterus in a 60 year old woman may no longer have the capacity to sustain growing fetal life. A 'normal' man does not have a uterus that can bear a child. 'Normal' life span differs for men and women, and differs between rich and poor countries. Thus, what is 'normal' changes from age to age, from culture to culture, and from sex to sex.

Shinn proposes that "the idea of normality... itself needs critical investigation."[37] Susan Wolf would concur. Wolf describes a danger that she calls "geneticism."[38] The danger is not genetic discrimination *per se.* Discrimination assumes that it acceptable to have a norm, but not to treat people differently when they fit the norm: if two of us are equally intelligent, one of us should not be denied education simply because she is female. This is discrimination. But the real danger, in Wolf's view, is not discrimination. It is 'geneticism.' It is the establishment of the (genetic) norms in the first place. It is the assumption that we can find a normatively 'human' and use it to decide who is deviant and needs to be 'corrected.' As Laurie Zoloth Dorfman suggests, "What the science of genetics has historically done is to frame the questions in the language of the dominant culture, and the questions themselves...carry the power to define personhood or, rather, successful personhood."[39]

Virgil's fiancee, out of her love for him, wanted to expand his possibilities, give him a new world, a 'seeing' world. No doubt she thought that life would be easier for Virgil if he could simply fit into the seeing world. She *assumed* that seeing is the norm and that Virgil would be a more successful person and better off if he could see. Her intentions were good. This alone should give us pause! Virgil's fiancee wanted Virgil to fit into *her* world; there is no suggestion that she considered blinding herself so as to fit into Virgil's world. This last suggestion is not as bizarre as it may seem. In a blind world, would a one-eyed man be 'king,' or would a one-eyed man need to be blinded so as to become 'normal'? If normal means 'usual,' then being deaf or blind might indeed be 'normal' in some communities and under some circumstances.

The danger, however, is that this will not be seen to be the case. Rather, the dominant community will impose its definition of 'normalcy' on other communities, seeking to 'correct' all those things which deviate from the norm. The imposition of definitions of normalcy will always reflect the views and experience of the dominant community. Since women and members of groups who are different but not powerful are never the dominant communities, we stand to lose in a 'geneticized' world.

Implications for justice

The imposition of standards that impose a definition from one culture onto another might be called 'cultural imperialism.' Cultural imperialism is one of the many faces of injustice identified by Iris Marion Young in her study of *Justice and the Politics of Difference.*[40]

Young argues that we are often if not always treated as members of 'groups' and that any theory of justice must take into account such group membership. A group is not simply an affiliation of people. It is not, for example, a lobby group or interest group. Rather, in Young's view, a morally relevant group is a social unit that has a shared history of oppression or privilege and a shared culture and way of doing things. A morally relevant group is "a collective of people who have affinity with one another because of a set of practices or way of life; they...are differentiated... according to these cultural forms."[41] In this sense, blind or deaf people might indeed form a 'group' in the relevant sense. They have a shared history of exclusion and oppression, and shared ways of doing things that are considered by others to be adaptations to the absence of vision or hearing, but in fact are simply how they learn to know and cope with the world. They are differentiated by such cultural forms.[42]

Moreover, they have experienced discrimination and oppression because of that differentiation. Among those forms of discrimination and oppression is cultural imperialism, the imposition of a norm derived from the dominant culture. Thus, deaf children are considered disabled, though the Deaf community does not agree.

Justice requires the redress of such forms of oppression. Young proposes that justice demands that such morally relevant social groups be given veto power over social policies that significantly affect them.[43] This suggests that learning what different groups want would be crucial to the establishment of justice in gene therapy. For example, the Little People of America would likely veto gene therapy for short stature except in cases where dwarfism is fatal. The Deaf community would veto gene therapy to correct deafness, though the Usher's community might allow therapy to prevent blindness. If justice requires that oppressed groups be given veto power, then some forms of gene therapy might not be universally acceptable, even for conditions that represent significant deviations from species-typical functioning.[44]

Yet Young's proposal is also not without its ambiguities. Who constitutes a 'group' in the morally relevant sense? Since not all deaf people are part of Deaf community, and since the morally relevant group is not to be simply identified with political lobby groups, who speaks for the deaf? Some deaf people *do* accept the definition of deafness as a disability;[45] whose view would be accepted, then, to represent the veto power of the morally relevant group?

Second, what are we to do when there is no well organized politically active group? Where there is a well organized group such as the Deaf or the Little People, it seems that the views of that group might prevail. However, the presence of an organized community may make the Deaf community or Little People different from other groups of people who have deviations from species-typical functioning, such as Tourette's or blindness. Increasingly, groups who are different from the statistical norm but do not consider themselves disabled are forming political communities and arguing that they are not disabled and do not need to be 'fixed.'[46] But not all people with disabilities have disability-identified groups who are well organized politically. Virgil belonged to no active 'disability rights' group or well organized political group. Should the absence of a well-organized and politicized group render some people with differences vulnerable to interventions that others might avoid? Should not the same protections be available to all those with differences who are distinguishable as a 'group' in a morally relevant sense? As tempting as Young's proposal is, there would be problems in practice with identifying morally relevant groups and their spokes people.

Nonetheless, Young's proposal points us toward the fundamental justice issue: the imposition of cultural standards on those who are different may in fact be oppressive rather than liberatory. That means that what the dominant majority considers 'therapy' is not always unambiguously good, but can be problematic. Perhaps the real question is, What would it mean to imagine a society without disabilities? Would it mean that every abnormality caused by a genetic deviation would be subjected to gene therapy? Or would it mean that social adaptations would render such abnormalities non-disabling? As Susan Wendell puts it, "When I imagine a society without disabilities, I do not imagine a society in which every physical and mental 'defect' or 'abnormality' can be cured.... Instead, I imagine a fully accessible society, the most fundamental characteristic of which is universal recognition that all structures have to be built and all activities have to be organized for the widest possible range of human abilities."[47] Too quick a move to gene 'therapy' may blind us to seeing the requirements of justice and honoring the perspectives of those who are different. Justice requires not an easy and universal acceptance of gene therapy, but precisely a deep and uneasy questioning of the very norms that undergird presumably therapeutic practices.

These reflections should not be taken to mean that gene therapy is wrong. Rather, they present some weighty cautions. First, what is 'therapy' to the dominant group may be an unwarranted intervention to marginalized groups; justice requires that the views of marginalized groups be taken seriously. Second, even where intervention might be welcomed or accepted, its effects may be more ambiguous than anticipated. Preparation is needed for interventions, and some interventions that bring good will also bring results that are perceived as bad. Third, there is a danger in the term 'therapy' itself. It is a seductive term that can lull us into thinking that there are no problems. In fact, however, the very establishment of a norm, the presumption that we know what needs to be 'fixed,' and the ambiguities of intervention are problematic. Thus, a shift from the language of gene therapy to the language of genetic intervention may be in order.

Notes

1. As told by neurologist Oliver Sacks, 1995, pp. 108–152.
2. A similar phenomenon appears to occur in children who are implanted with cochlear implants. Even if the child was previously hearing, the cochlear implant does not necessarily restore meaningful hearing. See Lane, 1993, pp. 218–224.
3. Sacks, 1995, p. 152.
4. Ibid., p. 151. Virgil, too, developed symptoms that are often associated with depression, such as extreme weight gain, and also became severely ill.
5. Language itself betrays me here. It is necessary to use a term such as 'disability', but in fact one of the issues at stake is precisely whether every difference is really a disability and what it means to call something a disability. I will return to this below.
6. See e.g. Walters, Palmer, 1997, p. 72. In a recent review of gene therapy studies, Kathleen Glass et.al. list a number of potential problems: contamination of the vector resulting in transfer of an unwanted gene or administration of a competent virus; the triggering of an immune response; interruption of the host's tumor suppressor genes; risk of infection of others with viruses; etc. See Glass et. al., 1999.
7. One of the most vexing issues is how to define disability. Most commentators (e.g., Bickenbach, 1993) adopt the United Nations distinction that *impairment* is a loss or abnormality of anatomical structure or function; *disability* is restriction or lack of ability to perform an activity considered normal for a human; and *handicap* is the disadvantage resulting for a person from either impairment or disability. However, philosopher Susan Wendell is critical of the UN definition. See Wendell, 1996, p. 14.
8. Walters, Palmer, 1997, p. 38; emphasis added.
9. Thompson, 1994, Chapter 1.
10. Lebacqz, 1996, pp. 3–14.
11. I use 'deaf' to indicate someone without hearing, and 'Deaf' to indicate someone who belongs to the community of people who do not take deafness to be a disability, but simply a cultural difference.
12. Sacks suggests that when deaf people are rendered Hearing (through cochlear implants, for example), they lose their identity, and that this identity is not simply a matter of being deaf but of belonging to a community with its own history, language, and culture. See Sacks, 1995, p. 142.

13. Lane, 1993, p. 5.
14. Harlan Lane tells a charming story of a little boy who was deaf and became friendly with the little girl next door; when she failed to understand his intricate hand gestures (his speech), he went to his mother and asked her what the other child's affliction was. His mother explained that the child did not know how to Sign. Lane, 1993, p. 92.
15. See for example Dolnick, 1993, pp. 37–53.
16. For example, Robert Van Etten is quoted as saying, "If there were a magic pill that would make me wake up tomorrow and be tall, I would not take it. Height has made me what I am." See Berreby, p.16. The official position of the Little People of America as found on their Web page is nuanced: they accept genetic intervention to prevent instances of dwarfism that cause death or serious other medical problems, but not simply to prevent short stature. See "Do We Really Want This?: Little People of America Inc. Comes to Terms with Genetic Testing," 1995. See www.lpaonline.org (Little People of America online).
17. These quotes are taken from a pamphlet prepared by the Ecumenical Working Group on Faith and Genetics for the 1998 Ecumenical Roundtable on Science, Technology and the Church in the U.S. and Canada, April 23, 1998.
18. Entitled "The Ragin' Cajun," this show has been aired on Public Broadcasting System several times. Usher's syndrome is particularly prevalent in a community whose origins were French, who settled in Nova Scotia and were evicted by the British, moving then to French Louisiana (hence, 'cajun' country), and now many of whom live outside Seattle. "The Ragin' Cajun" is the name of a restaurant opened by one young man with Usher's syndrome.
19. See, e.g. Lane, 1993, p. 14.
20. Sacks tells the story of a surgeon with Tourette's syndrome in "A Surgeon's Life," 1995, pp. 77–107. Dr. Carl Bennett was married with two children and a very well respected surgeon whose bizarre outbursts and compulsive behavior completely subsided when he did surgery. For a novel that tells the story of a young woman with Tourette's, see Rubio, 1998.
21. See, for example, members.tripod.com/~tourette13; also www.citynet.net/personal/chad.
22. Sacks, 1970, pp. 92–101.
23. Ibid., p. 98.
24. Wendell, 1996, p.78.
25. Ibid., 1996, p. 26. Wendell contracted myalgic encephalomyelitis (chronic fatigue syndrome) in 1985 and has lived with constant pain and fatigue ever since.
26. Ibid., 1996, p. 65.
27. Ibid., 1996, p. 19 notes that aging is disabling in almost all societies, and that therefore those who think of themselves as non-disabled are only so temporarily!
28. Sacks, 1970, p. 99.
29. In his later work (*An Anthropologist on Mars*), Sacks still describes Tourette's as a disorder (p. 84), but also acknowledges that there may be a 'normal' in Tourette's that simply differs from our 'normal' (p. 97).
30. Wendell, 1996, p. 24. Lane makes this point powerfully as well in The Mask of Benevolence, noting that "to portray a group is to engage in a political activity" (p. 69).
31. Ibid., p. 37. Similarly, Barbara Hillyer notes that our strong social ethic of productivity has very serious implications for people with disabilities and for those who care for them. See Hillyer, 1993.
32. Ibid., p. 42.
33. It is ironic that the movement to argue for the language of difference rather than disability is called the 'disability rights' movement.
34. For example, Barbara Hillyer argues that we must not neglect the very real problems that some people have, and that the language of 'difference' tends to mask the need for services. Hillyer, 1993, p. 28. Elsewhere (p.22) Hillyer says that each word pertaining to disability (difference, disability, handicap, able-ism, etc.) is a potential trap. I concur!
35. Laqueur, 1990.
36. Shinn, 1996, p. 96.
37. Ibid., p. 100f.
38. Wolf, 1995, pp. 345–53.
39. Zoloth Dorfman, 1998, p. 187.

40. Young, 1990. Young distinguishes five 'faces' of oppression: exploitation, marginalization, powerlessness, violence, and cultural imperialism.
41. Ibid., p. 186.
42. For example, Wendell claims that "from medical and rehabilitative practitioners' point of view..., a deaf child is disabled in her inability to hear.... But from another, equally valid point of view, the same child [is not disabled but simply] is handicapped by hearing people's...ignorance of Sign." Wendell,1996, p. 29.
43. Young, 1990, p. 184. Of course, determining the boundaries of relevant groups will be very difficult. See Lebacqz, 1998.
44. This view that would give groups veto power stands in direct contradiction to the dominant American view, clearly expressed in the work of John Robertson (see, e.g., *Children of Choice: Freedom and the New Reproductive Technologies*, 1994). Robertson argues that individuals have a right of reproductive liberty that encompasses the right to use any technologies necessary to choose the characteristics of their children.
45. See, for instance, Tucker, 1998, pp. 6–14.
46. For example, I have argued elsewhere that the emergence of the Intersex Society of North America (ISNA) may be crucial for assisting people born with ambiguous genitals to assert their identity as different rather than disabled. See Lebacqz, 1997, pp. 213–229.
47. Wendell, 1996, p. 55.

Bibliography

Berreby, D. 1996. "Up with People", *The New Republic* April 29, pp.15–19.

Bickenbach, J. E., 1993. *Physical Disability and Social Policy.* University of Toronto Press: Toronto.

Dolnick, E., 1993. "Deafness as Culture." *The Atlantic Monthly* 272, 3, pp. 37–53.

Ecumenical Working Group on Faith and Genetics, 1998. 1998 Ecumenical Roundtable on Science, Technology and the Church in the U.S. and Canada, April 23.

Glass, K., et.al. 1999. "Structuring the Review of Human Genetics Protocols, Part III: Gene Therapy Studies." *IRB: A Review of Human Subjects Research* 21, 2 (March–April).

Hillyer, B., 1993. *Feminism and Disability.* University of Oklahoma Press: Norman OK.

Lane, H., 1993. *The Mask of Benevolence: Disabling the Deaf Community.* Vintage Books: New York.

Laqueur, T., 1990. *Making Sex: Body and Gender from the Greeks to Freud.* Harvard University Press: Cambridge MA.

Lebacqz, K., 1996. "Diversity, Disability, and Designer Genes: On What It Means to be Human." *Studia Theologica: Scandinavian Journal of Theology* 50, 1, pp. 3–14.

Lebacqz, K., 1997. "Difference or Defect?: Intersexuality and the Politics of Difference." *Annual of the Society of Christian Ethics* 17, pp. 213–229.

Lebacqz, K., 1998. "Difficult Difference." *Cambridge Quarterly of Healthcare Ethics* 7, 1 (Winter).

Robertson, J., 1994. *Children of Choice: Freedom and the New Reproductive Technologies*. Princeton University Press: Princeton.

Rubio, G. H., 1998. *Icy Sparks.* Viking Penguin: New York.

Sacks, O., 1970. "Witty, Ticcy Ray." In: *The Man Who Mistook His Wife for a Hat.* Harper and Row: New York, San Francisco, London.

Sacks, O., 1995. "To See and Not See." In: *An Anthropologist on Mars: Seven Paradoxical Tales*. Alfred A. Knopf: New York.

Shinn, R., 1996. *The New Genetics: Challenges for Science, Faith, and Politics*. Moyer Bell: Wakefield R.I.

Thompson, L. 1994. *Correcting the Code: Inventing the Cure for the Human Body.* Simon and Shuster: New York.

Tucker, B., 1998. "Deaf Culture, Cochlear Implants, and Elective Disability." *Hastings Center Report* 28, 4, pp. 6–14.

Walters, L., Palmer, J. G., 1997. *The Ethics of Human Gene Therapy.* Oxford University Press: New York.

Wendell, S., 1996. *The Rejected Body: Feminist Philosophical Reflections on Disability.* Routledge: New York.

Wolf, S. M., 1995. "Beyond 'Genetic Discrimination': Toward the Broader Harm of Geneticism." *Journal of Law, Medicine and Ethics* 23, pp. 345–53.

Young, I. M., 1990. *Justice and the Politics of Difference*. Princeton U. Press: Princeton N. J.

Zoloth Dorfman, L., 1998. "Mapping the Normal Human Self: The Jew and the Mark of Otherness." In: Peters, T. (ed.). *Genetics: Issues of Social Justice*. The Pilgrim Press: Cleveland, OH.

ERIC T. JUENGST

Anticipating Enhancement: A Conceptual and Ethical Challenge for Gene Therapy Regulation

Introduction

The foundation for the public regulation of human gene therapy in most countries is a simple four-celled matrix of policy-relevant considerations. The matrix is created by crossing the two possible kinds of cellular targets for human gene transfer—somatic or germ-line cells—with the two possible goals one might have in performing it: treatment for disease or human "enhancement."[1] Both distinctions are widely debated, but in practice they have been crucial to human gene transfer research by creating the boundaries that protect the one form of human gene transfer that we are scientifically ready to pursue: somatic cell gene transfer interventions aimed at treating disease. As long as social policy decisions regarding germ-line and enhancement uses of gene transfer techniques could be postponed through provisional prohibitions, attention could be directed to regulating the proper conduct of somatic cell gene transfer as a new example of traditional medicine. Increasingly, however, policy-makers are being asked to directly address these boundaries, in anticipation of scientific advances. Much of that recent literature, has been focused on the line between somatic cell and germ-line gene therapy.[2] But while the somatic/germ-line distinction is accused of lacking adequate ethical force,[3] the conceptual line it draws is at least clear. The treatment/enhancement distinction, on the other hand, often seems in danger of evaporating entirely under conceptual critiques even before the question of its moral merits is entertained. If "enhancement" is to keep serving as a major policy boundary, we should at least be clear about just what it demarcates. My primary goal in this essay is to undertake that clarification. I will argue that, while there are a number of interpretations of "enhancement" available to policy makers, the ones that most accurately identify the public policy interests at stake in human gene transfer research are those that focus on the uses of gene transfer that would serve to exacerbate, rather than reform, the social injustices that flow from our intolerance for human biological variation.

The treatment/enhancement distinction

The treatment-enhancement distinction is usually used to argue that curative or therapeutic uses of genetic engineering fall within (and are protected by) the boundaries of medicine's traditional domain, while enhancement uses do not, and to that extent are more problematic as a professional medical practice or a legitimate health care need.[4] Unfortunately, making the distinction between treatment and enhancement is not without its own complexities. The distinction is explicated in at least three distinctly different ways, which have different merits as boundary markers for medical research and practice. There are accounts that rely on medicine's own understanding of its professional goals, accounts which rely on theoretical measures of "species-typical functioning" that go well beyond medicine, and accounts that turn on particular concepts of disease.

Professional domain accounts

One approach to the enhancement/treatment distinction is to define it in terms of the accepted limits of professional medical practice. Under this view, "treatments" are any interventions which physicians and their patients agree are useful and proper, while "enhancements" are simply interventions which are considered to fall beyond a physician's professional purview. Thus, physician-prescribed physical therapy to improve muscle strength would be considered legitimate medical treatment, while weight-lifting under a coach's supervision to achieve a particular physique would be considered an enhancement. This view resonates well with a number of contemporary social scientific critiques of biomedicine, which suggest that medicine has no natural domain of practice beyond that which it negotiates with society.[5] It also provides a simple normative lesson for professionals concerned about their obligations in specific cases: One takes one's cues from the patient's value system, and negotiates towards interventions that can help achieve the patient's vision of human flourishing.[6]

Unfortunately, however, these same features also deny this approach the ability to be of help to those attempting to use the treatment/enhancement distinction in order to regulate gene transfer research. Relying on the conventions of professional practice provides no principled way to classify technological innovations as either within or outside medicine's proper domain until after the fact of their acceptance or rejection by the medical community. To the extent that useful "upper-boundary" concepts are required at the policy level—for societies making health care research allocation decisions, for example—this impotence is an important weakness.

Normalcy accounts

Fortunately, another approach to interpreting the treatment/enhancement distinction is framed explicitly as a policy tool for separating legitimate health care needs from luxury services. The most developed exposition of this view is Sabin and Daniels endorsement of what they call the "normal function" standard for determining the limits of "medically necessary" (and therefore socially underwritten) mental health services.[7] Sabin and Daniels argue that an appropriate boundary between medically necessary treatments and optional enhancements line can be drawn simply by thinking about how to provide medical services fairly within a population. Following Daniels' earlier work,[8] they construe health care as one of society's means for preserving equality of opportunity for its citizens, and define health care needs as those services that allow individuals to enjoy the portion of the society's "normal opportunity range" to which their full array of skills and talents would give them access, by restoring or improving their abilities to the range of functional capacities typical for members of their reference class (e.g., age and gender) within the human species. Daniels has specified this definition of health care needs further by saying that the notion of "species-typical functioning" it relies upon is not "merely a statistical notion," but implies "a theoretical account of the design of the organism," that describes the "natural functional organization of a typical member of the species." Any interventions that would take expand an individual's range of functional capacities beyond the range typical for his or her reference class would count as an (medically unnecessary) enhancement. Thus, Sabin and Daniels write:

> Treating illness and enhancing human capabilities may both be desirable social goals, but they should not be confused with one another. The normal function model holds that health care insurance coverage should be restricted to disadvantages caused by disease and disability unless society explicitly decides to use it to mitigate other forms of disadvantage as well.[9]

The "normal function" approach is a sophisticated attempt to define the limits of social obligations to provide health services for policy purposes, and comes close to accurately reconstructing the rationale behind many actual "line drawing" judgments by health care coverage plans and professional societies. Unfortunately, this approach is also semi-permeable in an important way for our purposes.

The first serious problem is the problem of prevention. While efforts at generic "health promotion" straddle the border of biomedicine, efforts to prevent the manifestation of specific maladies in individuals people are always accepted as legitimate parts of biomedicine, and would be automatically located on the "treatment" side of the enhancement boundary. On the other hand, one of the ways one can prevent a disease is to strengthen the body's ability to resist it long before any diagnosable problem appears. These forms of prevention all attempt to elevate bodily functions above the normal range, and to that extent seem to slide into enhancement. Consider the case that LeRoy Walters and Julie Palmer make for including some genetic enhancements within the domain of legitimate medical needs. They start with the paradigm of a non-genetic preventive intervention—immunization against infectious disease—and then drive their genetic truck through the border-crossing it creates:

> In current medical practice, the best example of a widely-accepted health-related physical enhancement is immunization against infectious disease. With immunizations against diseases like polio or hepatitis B, what we are saying is in effect, "The immune system that we inherited from our parents may not be adequate to ward off certain viruses if we are exposed to them. Therefore, we will enhance the capabilities of our immune system by priming it to fight against these viruses." From the current practice of immunizations against particular diseases, it would seem to be only a small step to try to enhance the general function of the immune system by genetic means. ... In our view, the genetic enhancement of immune system function would be morally justifiable if this kind of enhancement assisted in preventing disease and did not cause offsetting harms to the people treated by the technique.[10]

This argument is bolstered by the fact that the technical prospects for such preventive-enhancement interventions already look good, given gene therapy research now underway to treat ill patients in just those ways. Thus, gene therapist summarizes the prospects for using gene therapy in oncology this way:

> Over the next few years, it appears that the greatest application will be in the treatment of cancer, where a number of genes that have been isolated have the potential to *empower* the immune system to eliminate cancer cells... Human gene therapy cancer trials have also been initiated for insertion of the tumor necrosis factor (TNF) gene into T-lymphocytes in an effort *to enhance the ability* of T-lymphocytes to kill tumors. Another approach has been to insert the TNF gene into tumor cells in an effort *to induce a more vigorous immune response* against the tumor.[11]

Another gene therapy protocol already underway "treats" people with an inherited high risk of heart disease by increasing the number of low density lipoprotein receptors their blood cells carry, enhancing their ability to clear their high levels of cholesterol from their blood before it causes heart disease.[12] If it works to reduce their risk of heart disease, why not use it prophylacticly to reduce my more modest risk? Moreover, if human gene therapy protocols like these are acceptable as forms of preventive medicine, the critics ask, how can we claim that we should be "drawing the line" at enhancement?

Disease-based accounts

Probably the most common rejoinder to the problem of prevention is to distinquish the problems to which they respond. Treatments are interventions which address the health problems created by diseases and disabilities—"maladies" in the helpful language of Clouser, Culver and Gert (1981). Enhancements, on the other hand, are interventions aimed at healthy systems and normal traits. Thus, prescribing biosynthetic growth hormone to rectify a diagnosable growth hormone deficiency is legitimate treatment, while prescribing it for patients with normal growth hormone levels would be an attempt at "positive gene therapy" or enhancement.[13] On this account, to justify an intervention as appropriate medicine means to be able to identify a pathological problem in the patient; if no medically recognizable malady can be diagnosed, the intervention cannot be "medically necessary," and is thus suspect as an enhancement.

This interpretation has the advantages of being simple, intuitively appealing, and consistent with a good bit of biomedical behavior. Maladies are objectively observable phenomena and the traditional target of medical intervention. We can know maladies through diagnosis, and we can tell that we've gone beyond medicine when no pathology can be identified.[14] Thus, the pediatric endocrinologists discourage the enhancement uses of biosynthetic growth hormone by citing the old adage "If it ain't broke, don't fix it."[15] This interpretation is also the one at work in the efforts of professionals working at the boundary, like cosmetic surgeons, to justify their services in terms of relieving "diagnosable" psychological suffering rather than satisfying the aesthetic tastes of their clients,[16] and in our insurance companies' insistence on being provided with that diagnosis before providing coverage for such surgeries.

Unfortunately, this interpretation does also face at least two major difficulties. The first problem that any disease-based interpretation of the enhancement boundary faces is, of course, biomedicine's infamous nosological elasticity. It is not that hard to coin new maladies for the purposes of justifying the use of enhancement interventions. By interpreting the boundary of medicine in terms of maladies, this approach puts the power for drawing that boundary squarely in the profession's hands, with the corresponding potential for abuse. Moreover, the preventive powers of a give enhancement intervention can be difficult to disprove, if the targeted disease never manifests itself. Enhancing interventions would have the advantage of the man who claimed his dance was keeping dragons out of Central Park: until a dragon lands it is hard to argue that he's not providing a preventive service.

The more important problem, however, is that for practical purposes no matter how the line is drawn, most of the gene transfer interventions that could become problematic as enhancement interventions would not have to cross that line in order to be developed and approved for clinical use, because they will also have legitimate therapeutic applications.

In fact, most gene transfer protocols with potential for enhancement uses will first emerge as therapeutic agents. General cognitive enhancement interventions, for example, are likely to be approved for use only in patients with neurological diseases.[17] However, to the extent that they are in high demand by individuals who are merely suffering the effects of normal aging, the risk of unapproved or "off-label" uses of these products will be high.[18] This risk poses unique regulatory challenges. Even if, for example, the U.S. Food and Drug Administration (FDA) vigorously attempted to regulate genetic enhancement technology, under its current legislative mandate the agency is unlikely to regulate off-label uses of approved products.[19] Moreover, given the current regulatory vacuum surrounding the private practice of reproductive medicine, there is little to prohibit the application of these techniques to early human embryos as well, in hopes of effecting germ-line transformations.

This last point is critical for policy purposes, because it suggests that, in countries like the U.S.A., the real challenge to regulation in this area may not be the development of enhancement interventions or "enhancement research" but about the downstream "off-label" uses of gene therapies for non-medical enhancement purposes. The policy problems then becomes one of controlling access and use of the technologies, not their research and development. Under the current policies of the U.S. FDA, for example, the discoverers of genetic enhancements have little incentive to even seek FDA approval for the enhancement uses of the therapeutic products. Obtaining approval of an enhancement claim, presumably in the form of an approved SNDA would require submission of the results of expensive clinical investigations. Even then, the fate of an SNDA would be uncertain, since the FDA lacks the experience and expertise to evaluation the safety and efficacy of enhancement technologies, particularly in view of the intangible and subjective nature of enhancement benefits.[20]

In addition, manufacturers have less likelihood of being liable under products liability law for injuries caused by the off-label uses of their products than for approved uses. While the courts are split on the subject, at least several have declined to hold a manufacturer liable for off-label injuries due to the "learned intermediary doctrine", which places the responsibility on the physician to assure the safety of off-label uses that the physician prescribes.[21] Unless the law is changed, regulation of genetic enhancements under the common law—which, given the absence of FDA regulation of off-label uses remains the most potent potential source of legal regulation—will focus on physician malpractice and actions for lack of informed consent. This presents another set of challenges for the law, since the novelty of genetic enhancement technologies will make it difficult for judges and juries to ascertain the reasonableness of physician behavior.

These realities have pressed those who would use the treatment/enhancement distinction for policy purposes to articulate the moral dangers of genetic enhancement more clearly.[22] After all, personal improvement is praised in many spheres of human endeavor, and, as purely elective matter, biomedical interventions like cosmetic surgery are well accepted in our society as means to achieving personal improvement goals.

Enhancement as a form of cheating

There are two lines of thought that have emerged from this recent work. The first focuses on the idea that biomedical enhancements are a form of social cheating. This is the view that taking the biomedical short-cut erodes the specific social practices that would make the analogous human achievement valuable in the first place. Thus, some argue that it defeats the purpose of the contest for the marathon runner to gain endurance chemically rather than through training, and it misses the point of meditation to gain Nirvana through psychosurgery. In both cases, the value of the improvements lie in the achievements they reward as well as the benefits they bring. The achievements—successful training or disciplined meditation—add value to the improvements because they are understood to be admirable social practices in themselves. Wherever a biomedical intervention is used to by-pass an admirable social practice, then, the improvement's social value—the value of a runner's physical endurance or a mystic's visions—is weakened accordingly. If we are to preserve the value of the social practices we count as "enhancing," it may be in society's interest to impose a means-based limit on biomedical enhancement efforts.

Interpreting enhancement interventions as those which short-circuit admirable human practices has special utility for policy analysis. To the extent that biomedical shortcuts increasingly allow specific accomplishments to be divorced from the admirable practices they were designed to signal, the social value of those accomplishments will be undermined. Not only will the intrinsic value be diminished for everyone that takes the short-cut, but the resulting disparity between the enhanced and unenhanced will call the fairness of the whole game (be it educational, recreational or professional) into question. If the extrinsic value of being causally responsible for certain accomplishments is high enough (like professional sports salaries), the intrinsic value of the admirable practices that a particular institution was designed to foster may even start to be called into question.[23] For institutions interested in continuing to foster the social values for which they have traditionally been the guardians, this has two alternative policy implications. Either they must redesign the game (of education, sports, etc.) to find new ways to evaluate excellence in the admirable practices that are not affected by available enhancements, or they must prohibit the use of the enhancing short-cuts. Which route an institution should take depends on the possibility and practicality of taking either, because ethically they are equivalent.

One of the reasons why pre-implantation genetic enhancements are more controversial than other forms of enhancement intervention is that they would be performed at a stage of human development that would allow the intervention to affect all the tissues in the body, including the germ-line cells. Enhancement interventions at this stage would either involve gene transfers or cell hybridizations performed with early human embryos conceived in vitro. These techniques are being improved steadily by molecular biologists in the production of "transgenic" animals for research purposes, and could some day be used to attempt to cure genetic diseases that begin their pathogenesis early in human development. That prospect, of introducing inheritable genetic changes through "germ-line gene therapy," is itself quite controversial, of course. However, since most couples willing to entertain germ-line gene therapy to prevent transmitting their genetic risks would also accept pre-implantation screening and selective embryo transfer to achieve that goal, it may be that the main practical rationale for using these techniques in humans will be for enhancement purposes.

In the U.S., moreover, this risk is exacerbated by the fact that, as this research moves from animal models to human experimentation, the long standing federal ban on human embryo research will force it to leave the hands of federally funded scientists with an interest in focusing their work on therapeutic applications, and move into the private world of infertility specialists, whose research efforts are not required to meet the same level of public accountability and review.[24] In that environment, which the client-centered ethos of reproductive medicine already imbues with a heavy interest in accommodating the reproductive goals of (paying) clients, the prospect of developing pre-implantation genetic enhancement interventions could become palatable long before it would in more traditional biomedical settings, and research towards that end could proceed without the national oversight that actual gene therapy research would require.[25] Thus, even before we engage the debate over the safety and propriety of human germ-line modification per se, the regulation of research and clinical innovation in reproductive medicine will become a critical challenge for those interested in developing responsible social policy regarding genetic enhancement.

Enhancement as an abuse of medicine

Unfortunately, some of the social games we can play (and cheat in) do not turn on participants' achievements at all, but on traits over which individuals have little control, like stature, shape and skin color. The social games of stigmatization, discrimination and exclusion use these traits in the same manner that other practices use achievements: as intrinsically valuable keys to extrinsic goods. Now it is becoming increasingly possible to seek biomedical help in changing these traits in order to short circuit these games as well. Here, the biomedical interventions involved, like skin lighteners or stature increasers, are "enhancements" because they serve to improve the recipient's social standing, but only by perpetuating the social bias under which they originally labored. When "enhancement" is understood in this way, it warns of still another set of moral concerns.

On this interpretation, what makes the provision of human growth hormone to a short child a morally suspicious enhancement is not the absence of a diagnosable disease or the "species atypical" hormone level that would result: rather it is the intent to improve the child's social status by changing the child rather than by changing her social environment.[26] Enhancement interventions are almost always wrong-headed under this account, because the source of the social status they seek to improve is, by definition, the social group and not the individual. Attempting to improve that status in the individual amounts to a moral mistake akin to "blaming the victim:" it misattributes causality, is ultimately futile, and can have harmful consequences. This is the interpretation of enhancement that seems to be at work when people argue that it inappropriately "medicalizes" a social problem to use Ritalin to induce cooperative behavior in the classroom. In such cases, the critics dispute the assumption that the human need in question is one that is created by, and quenchable through, our bodies, and assert that both its source and solution really lie in quite a different sphere of human experience.

This interpretation of the enhancement concept is useful to those interested in the ethics of personal improvement because it warns of a number of moral pitfalls beyond the base-line considerations that the enhancement/treatment distinction provides. Attempting to improve social status by changing the individual risks being self-defeating (by inflating expectations), futile (if the individual's comparative gains are neutralized by the enhancement's availability to the whole social group) unfair (if the whole group does not have access to the enhancement) or complicitous with unjust social prejudices (by forcing people into a range of variation dictated by biases that favor one group over others). For those faced with decisions about whether to attempt to enhance themselves or their children through gene transfer, this way of understanding enhancement is much more illuminating than attempts to distinguishing it from medical treatment, because it points to the real values at stake. Ideally, one should do no gene transfer that will make an existing social problem worse, even if exacerbating injustice would further one's own interests.

On the other hand, protecting these values is difficult in a pluralistic society like ours, because it means developing ways to policing individuals' complicity with suspect social norms.[27] Under the historical shadow of state sponsored eugenics programs, our government is unlikely to promulgate lists of acceptable and unacceptable enhancements, even if the intent of the lists are to protect the interests of those who are unenhanced.

Moreover, regulatory limits on access to genetic enhancements in the United States could be ineffectual if individuals could obtain enhancements abroad. In the past, we have seen a number of examples of persons circumventing US laws to obtain medical care abroad, including seeking illegal abortions abroad prior to Roe v. Wade;[28] purchasing unapproved AIDS drugs, RU486, and other pharmaceuticals abroad and returning with them to the United States;[29] travelling to foreign countries to obtain infertility treatments that were illegal or unavailable in the United States.[30] Most nations' ability under domestic legal authority to control off-shore access is extremely limited. For example, U.S. federal law permits customs officers routinely to search people entering the country for contraband, without requiring a warrant or probable cause.[31] However, border controls would not be suitable for stopping persons who had obtained gene insertion technologies abroad. Even if they could be identified, what sanction would they be subjected to: being forced to reverse the procedure? Kept in permanent quarantine? Another approach would be to try to prevent people from travelling abroad in the first place in order to obtain contraband enhancements. Again, the U.S. arguably possesses the authority to restrict travel on grounds of national security.[32] Would obtaining enhancements abroad amount to such a threat? Even if it did, travel restrictions have been imposed on travel to specific countries; it would be virtually impossible to restrict travel to a country for a specific purpose, if travel were permitted for other purposes.

An alternative would be for nations to attempt to affect the availability of genetic enhancements abroad through treaties and other public international legal mechanisms, such as the authority of the United Nations and regional political entities like the European Economic Community and the Council of Europe. Yet international efforts require commitment by multiple governments and effective methods of enforcement. It is unclear that either of these conditions would be met universally enough to block international access to enhancements. Indeed, it is more likely that a government of an impoverished country would view trade in enhancements as an ideal means of attracting foreign exchange.

Conclusion

It is important to remember, of course, that the sorts of "enhancements" we envision in these discussions may never become technically possible to achieve: most of the interesting ones—intelligence, memory, beauty, stamina, strength—are complex traits influenced only remotely by many of our genes in collaboration. In practice, we may never have to worry about crossing the enhancement line towards those improvements. On the other hand, if we do develop safe and efficacious ways to strengthening the immune system, slowing cellular aging, and preventing disease, the issues raised by the "enhancement" concept—the problem of social cheating and the need to discourage complicity with unjust social bias—will have to be addressed in policy. In doing so, three features of the genetic enhancement's regulatory environment will pose special challenges: the problem of "off-label" uses of interventions approved for therapeutic use, the entrepreneurial ethos of contemporary reproductive medicine, and the prospect of international access to enhancement interventions developed elsewhere. Each of these are social policy problems whose intersections with genetics that have received negligible attention, but which will become increasingly crucial to address as genomic medicine matures.

Acknowledgments

The research conducted for this chapter was supported in part by NIH grant # R01 HG-1446-02. I am grateful to Tom Murray, Maxwell Mehlman, Erik Parens, and David Smith for useful discussions of the text and many of the ideas presented here.

Noter

1. Areen, 1985, Walters, 1986.
2. Cf. Resnick, Steinkraus, Langer, 1999.
3. Moseley, 1991.
4. Anderson, 1989, Baird, 1994.
5. Good, 1994.
6. Engelhardt, 1990.
7. Sabins, Daniels, 1994.
8. Daniels, 1986, 1992.
9. Sabin, Daniels, 1994.
10. Walters, Palmer, 1997, p.110.
11. Culver, 1993, emphasis added.
12. Wilson et al., 1992.
13. Berger, Gert, 1991.
14. Juengst, 1997.
15. Ad Hoc Committee, 1984.
16. Morgan, 1991.
17. Whitehouse et al., 1997.
18. Christopher, 1993.
19. Kessler, 1978.
20. Moertel, 1997.
21. Stoffelmayer, 1996
22. Parens, 1998.
23. Murray, 1984.
24. Byers, 1997.
25. Cohen, 1997.
26. White, 1993.
27. Little, 1998.

28. Kriemer, 1992.
29. Batterman, 1997.
30. Sauer, 1997.
31. 19 USC A7482, 1996.
32. Zemel v. Rusk, 381 US 1, 1965.

Bibliography

Ad Hoc Committee on Growth Hormone Usage, 1984. "Growth hormone in the treatment of children for short stature." *Pediatrics* 72, pp. 891–894.

Anderson, W. F., 1989. "Human gene therapy: Why draw a line?" *Journal of Medicine and Philosophy* 14, pp. 681–693.

Areen, J., 1985. "Regulating human gene therapy." *West Virginia Law Review* 88, pp. 153.

Baird, P., 1994. "Altering human genes: social, ethical and legal implications." *Perspectives in Biology and Medicine* 37, pp. 566–575.

Batterman, J. S., 1990. "Brother can you spare a drug?" *Hofstra University Law Review* 19, p. 191.

Berger, E., Gert, B. , 1991. "Genetic disorders and the ethical status of germ-line gene therapy." *Journal of Medicine and Philosophy* 16, pp. 667–685.

Byers, K., 1997. "A growing need for consumer-oriented regulation of the in vitro fertilization industry." *Journal of Legal Medicine* 18, 3, pp. 1–34.

Christopher, W., 1993. "Off-Label Drug Prescription: Filling the Regulatory Vacuum." *Food & Drug Law J.* 48, p. 247.

Clouser, K., Culver, C., Gert, B., 1981. "Malady: a new treatment of disease," *Hastings Center Report* 11, pp. 29–37.

Cohen, C., 1997. "Unmanaged care: The need to regulate new reproductive technologies in the United States." *Bioethics* 11, pp. 348–365.

Culver, K., 1993. "Current status of human gene therapy research." *The Genetic Resource* 7, pp. 5–10.

Daniels, N., 1986. *Just Health Care*. Cambridge University Press: New York.

Daniels, N. 1992. "Growth hormone therapy for short stature: can we support the treatment/enhancement distinction?" *Growth, Genetic and Hormones*, Suppl. 1, Vol. 8, pp. 46–48.

Engelhardt, H. T., 1990. "Human nature technologically revisited." *Social Philosophy and Policy* 8, pp. 180–191.

Good, B., 1994. *Medicine, Rationality and Experience: An Anthropological Perspective.* Cambridge University Press: New York.

Juengst, E., 1997. "Can enhancement be distinguished from prevention in genetic medicine?" *Journal of Medicine and Philosophy* 22, pp. 125–142.

Kessler, D., 1978. "Regulating the Prescribing of Human Drugs for Non-approved
Uses under the Food, Drug, and Cosmetic Act." *Harvard Journal on Legislation* 15, p. 693.

Kriemer, 1992. "The law of choice and the choice of law: Abortion, the right to travel and extraterritorial regulation in American federalism." *NYU Law Review* 67, p. 451.

Little, M., 1997. "Suspect norms of appearance and the ethics of complicity." In: de Beaufort, I., Hilhorst, M., Holm, S. (eds.). *In the Eye of the Beholder: Ethics and Medical Change of Appearance*. Scandinavian University Press: Oslo, pp. 151–167.

Moseley, R., 1991. "Maintaining the somatic/germ-line distinction: Some ethical drawbacks." *Journal of Medicine and Philosophy* 16, pp. 641–649.

Morgan, K., 1991. "Women and the knife: Cosmetic surgery and the colonization of women's bodies." *Hypatia* 6, pp. 25–53.

Moertel, C. G., 1991. "Off-Label Drug Use for Cancer Therapy and National Health Care Priorities." *JAMA* 266, p. 3031.

Murray, T. 1984. "Drugs, Sports and Ethics." In: Murray, T., Gaylin, W., Macklin, R. (eds.). *Feeling Good and Doing Better: Ethics and Nontherapeutic Drug Use*. Humana Press: Clifton NJ, pp. 107–129.

Parens, E. 1998. "Is better always good?" *The Hastings Center Report* 28, S1–S17.

Parens, E. 1995. "The goodness of fragility: On the prospect of genetic technologies aimed at the enhancement of human capabilities." *Kennedy Institute of Ethics Journal* 5, pp. 141–153.

Resnick, D., Steinkraus, H., Langer, P., 1999. *Human Germline Gene Therapy: Scientific, Moral and Political Issues*. R.G. Landes Co.: Austin, TX.

Sabin, J., Daniels, N., 1994. "Determining 'medical necessity' in mental health practice." *Hastings Center Report* 24, pp. 5–13.

Sauer, J., 1997. "Reproductive prohibition: Restricting donor payment will lead to medical tourism." *Human Reproduction* 12, pp. 1844–1845.

Stoffelmayer, K., 1996. "Products liability and "off-label" uses of prescriptions drugs." *University of Chicago Law Review* 63, p. 275.

Walters, L., 1986. "The Ethics of Human Gene Therapy." *Nature* 320, pp. 225–227.

Walters, L., Palmer, J., 1997. *The Ethics of Human Gene Therapy.* Oxford University Press: Oxford.

White, G., 1993. "Human growth hormone: The dilemma of expanded use in children." *Kennedy Institute of Ethics Journal* 3, pp. 401–409.

Whitehouse, P., Juengst, E., Murray, T., Mehlman, M., 1997. "Enhancing cognition in the intellectuallly intact." *Hastings Center Report* 27, 3, pp. 14–22.

Wilson J., et. al., 1992. "*Ex Vivo* gene therapy for familial hypercholesterolemia." *Human Gene Therapy* 3, pp. 179–222.

National Perspectives: Germany and Japan

DIETMAR MIETH

The Ethics of Gene Therapy: The German Debate

Introduction

In 1993 and 1994, the German *Bundesärztekammer* and a Commission or Advisory Group of the *Bund* (federation) and the *Länder* (federal states) cooperated in the regulation of gene therapy. The ethical questions were: how much regulation and what kind of regulation is necessary? Because the Guidelines of the *Bundesärztekammer* (January 1995) function like laws in medical experimentation on humans—in this case, clinical trials for gene therapy—there was until now no need for new laws. And it should be noted that since germ-line experimentation on human subjects is clearly prohibited in Germany by law, the regulations concern only somatic cell gene therapy.

There are some points which are specific for the German debate on gene therapy:

- the widespread lack of confidence in "bioethics" resulting from the so-called Singer debate on early euthanasia, the discussion about the (Bioethics) Convention of the Council of Europe, and the discussion of the UNESCO (Bioethics) Declaration on the Human Genome;
- the impact of ecology on religious or Christian movements, above all among grassroots activists within the Protestant church;
- the specific history of Germany, which requires sensitivity to phenomena like "selection" and the identification of individual subjects through genetic information;
- the context of the discussion about abortion, in which the eugenic indication (now hidden under the medical indication) entails a specific approach; the struggle between Pro-life groups and Pro-choice groups has an international context but is becoming stronger in Germany today; (conflict between Bavaria and the German Constitution Court);
- the consensus against germ-line manipulation which does not give social acceptance to certain abstract philosophical and even theological arguments in favor of germ-line cell gene therapy "in itself."

These points are, of course, more or less specific, but we can clearly see that each line of ethical argumentation has a particular German context.

My information about the specific debate on somatic cell gene therapy and clinical trials comes from two, admittedly incomplete, sources: the Guidelines of the *Bundesärztekammer* (BAK), reported in the minutes of the *Bund-Länder-Kommission*, and the survey by Traute M. Schröder-Kurth and her assistent, Janine E. Lunshof, in the book *Ethik und Gentherapie*.[1]

The regulation of somatic gene transfer is based on the *Berufsordnung für die deutschen Ärzte* (German Medical Professional Code), on the *Arzneimittelgesetz* (regulations governing the manufacture and prescription of drugs), and on the guidelines for medical ethics commissions. In the BAK Guidelines, the international standard of the discussion is repeated: "The application of somatic cell gene therapy evokes no ethical and juridical problems which are fundamentally new. As a method of molecular medicine it realizes the ends on a new level. In the adequate cases, this method is medically and ethically acceptable, insofar as there is enough guarantee for the technical and biological safety of the method of transfer and of the application of the rules of regulation for biomedical research on human beings" (2.3). On this basis, the *Bundesärztekammer* founded a new institution: the Central Commission on "Somatic Cell Gene Therapy." The exchange between local committees and the central committee is to be regulated by the principle of subsidiarity. The ethical commissions in medicine act as controlling advisory groups. They have no right to make decisions.

I will not go into the details of the medical approval of somatic gene therapy and its criteria. K.W. Schmidt gives a good summary of the criteria from an ethical perspective:[2]

1. The protection of the welfare and dignity of the patient;
2. Informed consent;
3. The safety of the trial;
4. A positive relationship between costs and benefits;
5. An indication of diseases following the criteria of justice;
6. The protection of data and the private spheres of patients;

This is surely not specific for the German debate. It is more typical for an international ethical agreement, even if the application of these criteria remains complicated in practice. But it is clear that even though somatic gene therapy is accepted by a great majority, the German debate involves fundamental conflict. The arguments of the opposition are discussed in the recent book on gene therapy by Ursel Fuchs, *Gentechnik, Der Griff nach dem Erbgut, Eine kritische Bestandsaufnahme*.[3] These arguments are:

1. Gene therapy has not been very successful thus far; it remains a utopia "in vivo."
2. We do not know the risks.[4]
3. Informed consent includes more than the consent to experimentation (for example, to proliferation of data and to further control).
4. There is economic pressure, because the therapies being tested or under development are products of commercial enterprises, some of which are under way of claiming patents.
5. Somatic cell gene therapy under strict ethical guidelines will not be very successful. As a result, it is only a step towards the acceptance of germ-line manipulation or selecting methods in genetic testing in vitro which are becoming increasingly important.

We can see the difference between the criteria of "bioethics" and the arguments of the opposition. However, I shall not elaborate on this discussion here. Instead, I shall focus on some more hermeneutic questions. In the following more systematic reflections, I shall take this difference into account.

Germ-line cell gene therapy

The strong global rejection of germ-line therapy has gradually been replaced by a highly differentiated discussion in bioethics. The categorical rejection assumes that we may refrain from applying possible therapies for widespread genetic/hereditary diseases because the status quo of genetic information, considered as "nature," is not permitted to be changed. Conversely, others assert our responsibility to offer therapy and our responsibility to future generations.

If we proceed from the categorical level to the level of evaluation, then the arguments for a legal ban predominate. However, the presuppositions of this juridical restraint may change, although this is somewhat improbable at present. The following reasons are often given against the approval of germ-line therapy:

- Research and development of germ-line therapy require exhaustive and exceedingly thorough experimentation on early embryos, experiments which, according to this opinion, are ethically intolerable. Should, however, the achievability of so-called "higher ranking goals" become plausible, the debate will undoubtedly be reopened, even in as restrictive a country as Germany.
- The isolation of the therapeutic experiment and thus of the effects is so difficult to carry out that ultimately unacceptable side effects are to be expected. There is no therapy which is "safe in itself."

- We should not reject the teleological argument that experimentation on the human genotype will lead to a complicated debate on a new definition of limits: What is disease? What constitutes a diseased or "unhealthy" gene? Does the individual interest, as is generally the case at the moment, determine the need for therapy? It is also possible to formulate this argument as a principle: a narrow definition of limits is preferable to a broader one if the broader definition of limits is unclear and difficult to implement.
- We do not know the results of the further evolution of humankind in a changing ecological context. How can we directly manipulate the human genome if we live in a changing world in which we have no exact prognoses about the effects of our engineering? The argument that we will only continue to do what we always have done is not convincing. In that case, we must show that our influence on the human phenotype and genotype in the past was beneficial. At the very least, a case-by-case approach is needed. There will be a distinction between things which we do unknowingly and things regarding which we know that there will be many uncertainties. And we know at the same time that our actions will have irreversible results.
- How can we ignore the informed consent of future generations if we want to include their rights (the rights of how many generations?)? To speak of rights which cannot be claimed by the persons involved is not impossible, but the question of who decides ends with the decision of the parents, a decision which can only be characterized as "paternalistic". All the problems involved in paternalism arise here in a highly intensified form. The responsibility of parenthood cannot—contrary to Sass[5]—be extended to numerous future generations.

There are some differences to be taken into account between the European Convention on Human Rights and Biomedicine and the more restrictive options in the German debate and in the EU Parliament. The difference in approach can be explained by some documents. In Article 13 of the Convention we read: "An intervention seeking to *modify the human genome* may only be undertaken for preventive, diagnostic or therapeutic purposes and only if its aim is not to introduce any modification in the genome of any descendents." Only the direct intention to modify the genome of descendents is forbidden. On the other hand, we read in an amendment of the EU Parliament to the 5. Framework Research Programme in Biotechnology: "No research activity which is liable to modify the human genetic heritage by manipulation of germ cells or manipulation of an other stage in embryonic development, which modification might become part of the genetic heritage, will take place under the present framework programme." This declaration refers not only to the intention but to all activity of modification. In the negotiations between the EU Parliament, the Commission and the Council of Ministers, a so-called "Common position" has been formulated (in November 1998). The Parliament's text is changed in the following way: "No research activity which modifies or is intended to modify genetic heritage of *human beings* by alteration of germ cells or by activity at any other stage in embryonic development and which can make such alterations heritable will be carried out under the present framework programme." This seems to be only a modification in the formulation. But every detail is important. That the formulation on modification is not as strict as before is not the main alteration. We have to be aware that the Parliament speaks of the modification of *human* genetic heritage, and that the new proposal speaks of the genetic heritage of *human beings*. In this kind of language politics, the notion of "human" includes all of the species, while the notion of a "*human being*," in the context of the European Convention, keeps the question open whether early embryos are included.

In finding that the proposed Common Position is not as strict as the amendment of the EU Parliament and that it is closer to the Convention, we can establish that there are options or conceptions which do not exlude the intervention on germ-line cells in all conceivable cases. In the more liberal conception, a modification is not in itself unacceptable. Those who defend this view follow the politics of restriction to restrictions. They may think about acts with double effects where a modification which involves the descendents takes place without being intended but is a side effect of a treatment. An example are 'conventional' treatments of cancer with laser which may influence the germ cells and consequently reproduction. Another example is the treatment of mitochondrial diseases by replacing the nucleus of an egg. A third example is embryo research without implanting the manipulated embryo into the uterus. It is clear that in the last case the German position is stricter due to the regulation of the Embryo Protection Law.

Defining the limits to a selective and manipulative intentionality in human genetics research is imperative. Here the possibility of self-determination would actually be affected as well as the dignity of the subjects involved.

Somatic cell gene therapy

The following reflections on the ethical evaluation of somatic cell gene therapy arose in answer to questions which the *Bund/Länder* forum on gene therapy directed to the ethicists. The first question was about the distinction between classical methods of therapy and somatic gene therapy in terms of the well-known principles of medical ethics: "autonomy, nonmaleficence, beneficence, and justice". Does somatic gene transfer raise any specific ethical problems?

I made a distinction between two different uses of the word "specific". In one sense, it means "exclusive," indicating that these kinds of problems do not exist outside the field of medical methods. In the other sense, it means "significant," without pretending that the problems are only related to this field. In this latter sense, we may have significant problems in somatic cell gene therapy, problems which are not entirely new but create a need for a new sensitivity in the regulation of conventional problems in human medical experimentation.

In the first sense ("exclusive") the ethically relevant problems are:

1. The question of internal safety (side effects on the germ-line);
2. The question of safety for future generations;
3. The question of therapy, prevention, and prediction in the case of mere dispositions for a disease;
4. The question of "genification" (Genifizierung), i.e. the reduction of diagnosis and therapy to an issue of genetics, the change of the paradigm of medicine from a more multifactorial approach to a single factor approach;
5. The possibility of manipulation of populations by means of individual consent and interest.

In the second sense ("significant") the ethically relevant problems are:

1. Nonmaleficence:
a. Harmlessness of clinical trials (experimentation on human subjects reviewed by ethics committees)
b. Possible undesirable side effects
c. Possible toxic effects of vectors
d. Immunological reactions of the recipients of the gene transfers
2. Autonomy:
a. (Non-)directive invitation of ill persons to be test subjects
b. A balance between autonomy and solidarity in the definition of "illness/disease" and "therapy"
c. Informed consent in experimental therapies
3. Beneficence
a. Has a personal support of test subjects been provided?
b. How are failures dealt with?
c. Have any unreasonable promises been made?
d. Is the information about risks sufficient?
4. Justice (Definition: Alike is to be treated alike, unlike unlike.)

With regard to the last point, problems of priority-setting and financing arise: How can we reconcile the right to basic medical care and hygiene (for example, in the Two Thirds World) with the promotion of peak technology? To what extent can we speak of "Western diseases", diseases that we must attempt to fight through prevention? To what degree does the extension of life through medical advances at the same time paradoxically imply constant regulation of the right to medical care as well as its progressive differentiation?

Many aspects of these issues are of a general and intercultural nature. What is really needed for the time being may be to intensify our discussions.

Note that these reflections are not directed against somatic gene therapy, but they help to determine the principles for undertaking it.

The second question directed to the ethicists by the *Bund/Länder* forum concerned the need of establishing a catalogue of indications. This question might be hypothetical because we must first have methods which can be clinically approved and applied. Only then it is possible to rank the severity of diseases and the effectivity of application, and weigh benefits against risks.

The third question concerned the need for ethics committees. Regarding this issue I agree with the principles of German regulation and insist on more institutions and positions for genetic counselling. No diagnosis and no experimentation without professionally established counselling! This is also a principle of the German Human Genetics Association and a principle of the last recommendation of the Group of Advisers on the Ethical Implications of Biotechnology (GAEIB) to the EC on prenatal diagnosis.

There are some promising somatic gene transfer trials, but we have not yet any clinically applicable, repeatable, and approved "therapies". This means that the word "therapy" is one of the ideologically misused words which appear in this context, not least in the case of "therapeutic" in vitro cloning.

The UNESCO Declaration adresses germ-line cell manipulation only indirectly (Article 24). It contains also one article (No. 8) which awards compensation to persons who suffer harm because of genetic intervention. This was intended as a warning to researchers to do something which could possibly result in someone in the third generation having a claim to compensation. However, this is a very weak way to present this topic, and it is contradicted by Article 12 which states the right of all to the "benefits" of genetic engineering.

This is also a well known "trick" in ethical debate: to say that all persons should have equal access to the advantages offered by the new technologies. This principle of *access* easily turns into a principle of coercion when, for example, it is suggested to developing nations that they should promote precisely this technology so that they, too, will have "equal access." Here we are also dealing with a question of cultural autonomy, i.e., a question concerning the extent to which these countries are able to draw their own conclusions about what they consider important and *which* technologies they want to have *what kind of* access to.

If we turn to the European Convention on Human Rights and Biomedicine, we find that while Article 13 does not explicitly mention germ-line intervention, it still mentions it indirectly. It is forbidden to intervene with the goal of passing on certain characteristics to the next generation. Clearly this is intended as a restriction on the goals. Yet gene transfers may very well be carried out without the primary goal of transmitting the results to future generations even though they may nonetheless have this as a side effect. Thus, the Convention contains only a weak prohibition of germ-line intervention.

A strong prohibition of germ-line gene therapy?

Now one may ask: are there any ethical arguments in favour of a stronger prohibition? While I do not have any categorical arguments against germ-line cell therapy, I do have some arguments that, in my opinion, are very strong, even though they are not completely independent of the circumstances.

The first argument is the uncertainty argument. It deals not only with risks but also with the uncertainty of the risk we are willing to accept when we do not have any previous knowledge of the interaction between genes and the environment, and when we can become experienced only by doing the very thing which is supposed to be the object of evaluation. This is a problem with all risk assessments. Thus, risk assessment is an indirect form of technology promotion. This is also a matter of politics of language. However, what I am concerned about here is the argument from uncertainty.

The second argument is the irreversibility of intervention on the germ-line. One of the important controllers of research working for the European Union is J. Quintanilha. He leads the group (ELSA) which examines the ethical, legal, and social issues raised by research projects in this field and also awards such projects. This group consists of 14 persons, 12 of whom are biologists, one is a philosopher, and one is a lawyer. The president is obviously also a biologist which raises the political question: to what extent do the biologists determine which ethical, legal and social problems are addressed by the group rather than the other way around, that the problems raised by biology determine what is to be clarified by ethicists, social researchers and lawyers? This is the situation in the European Union. Quintanilha is of the opinion that if we had the technical ability to develop germ-line cell therapies, then the result would also be reversible. He says that this technology is so complicated that if we were to achieve it, we would also be in a position to be able to reverse it.

A third argument which is put forward over and over again is that future generations cannot consent to this manipulation. There is a lack of "informed consent." It is possible, due to multiple functions of single genes, that a genetic intervention will not only result in advantages but also in certain disadvantages. Since ethicists have reached a general consensus that individuals in a democratic society should have the right to decide about advantages and disadvantages, this concern carries weight.

These three arguments form a sort of cable made of different cords, a "convergence argument" which judges germ-line cell therapy to be ethically unacceptable. However, I would like to emphasize that Article 24 of the UNESCO Declaration only indicates that germ-line gene therapy is a possible moral problem, and that the prohibition in the European Convention on Human Rights and Biomedicine is expressed only very weakly.

Moreover, Quintanilha, the leader of ELSA, is of the opinion that we in the strict sense socially determine our lives, that we have a set of designs for our social life, that we raise children in particular ways, that we nourish ourselves in particular ways, that we have a particular culture, and that we are dominated by this whole system of science, technology, and economy. We already do intervene significantly in what makes us human. We already do determine human life to a large extent. With this in mind, he offers this *social* design of our lives as a reason why we could also change the *natural* design by means of cloning and negative selection. This kind of an argument appears frequently in the bio-political ethics strategy: why should we refrain from doing that which is in line with options we no longer question?

The answer to this is clear: we have good ethical reasons to restrict determinism in social design. This is why we strive for ethical autonomy in two senses: free self-determination and free self-obligation, the unity of *autos* and *nomos*. Thus, we in no way commit ourselves "morally" to actual determinism. Ethics is critical towards social determinism.

We have seen that biopolitics gives ethics strategic significance yet at the same time reduces it to an enforcement strategy. In the ethics advisory groups, the relationship between biopolitics and ethics is in fact dominated by biopolitics. This is not good. Only when moral judgements are *pre*-political—which does not mean they must be *un*-political—will political ethics be ethics once again, and this has to be implemented before politics completely accommodates ethics to itself.

What kind of a social environment do we want to live in? Do we wish sexuality to become more and more a thing of the brain? In that case, we may no longer need the erotic processes connected with it. The end of love lyrics is also the end of children's safety in the love of their parents. We may replace them by laboratory work. Maybe it will eventually be possible to procreate without pleasure. The monks of early Christianity strove for this. Augustine, for example, was of the opinion that the new humanity would best be procreated by parents touching each other only with their elbows and without lust.

But do we want erotic and sensual sexuality? Do we want to have this sensual form of skin-experience connected with the reproduction of humanity? Do we insist that it is embedded in the continuity and intensity of the love-bond? Whoever insists that in propagation, birth and death there are cultural achievements which determine our idea of the good life is acting in a value conserving way. To be a value conservative does not mean that one cannot act in a structurally progressive way. Value conservatives do not want to give up the embeddedness of reproduction in a culture of love as skin-experience which in the past has given us so much aesthetic production, paintings, and poetry.

Regarding the question of social environment, how we want the future to be, Jürgen Habermas has pointed out that the development of law depends on which values people affirm in their social context.[6] If this is true, then we must cultivate and question these values. This in no way means that every advance must be rejected. Rather, it means that we should examine whether an advance can be shaped in agreement with cultural values that are worth preserving. The decision about which cultural values and norms are worth preserving becomes relevant only within the unfolding of the argument of human dignity (see above). Moral culture and moral reconstruction stands in a relationship of mutual interaction.

The Eeugenics argument

In relation to the methods of human genetics—genetic diagnosis, gene transfer, and cloning—the topic of "eugenics" is often raised. Obviously we are dealing here with an important point of reference in moral examination. Of course, the word "eugenics" originally had no ethical content, but a descriptive one. According to Francis Galton (1883), it has to do with the reconceptualization of inheritance as a statistical condition of populations and future generations.[7]

This reconceptualization can be used to support the idea of selection, negatively of the "bad", positively of the "good." The extent of its misuse is far-reaching, from the sterilization of the mentally ill (Indiana, 1907) to the extermination of "those unworthy to live". These selections were carried out for racist or public health reasons. One must differentiate eugenics from euphenics (influence only on the individual phenotype, for example by somatic gene transfer) and euthenics (influence on the environment and living conditions).[8]

Only eugenics has to do with influences which go beyond the individual. "Eugenics should concern itself with all conditions which can contribute to the cultivation of genetic characteristics in future generations and to the development of those genetic assets in the lives of individuals which can contribute to the benefit of the whole."[9]

Let us focus on the notion of "benefit of the whole" which is also known as the "gene pool" argument. The assumption here is that the human genome is a "heritage of Humanity" (cf. the UNESCO Declaration) which can be influenced by human intervention. There are two possiblities: genetic degeneration (caused by, for example, human influences in terms of environmental degradation, misuse, or accidents) and genetic improvement (also caused by human intervention). At the scientific level, there is disagreement on whether it is possible to remove the arbitrariness of the genetic influences on populations and instead direct them. In general, this will hardly be possible, but in individual cases the reparation of burdens, i.e. genetic diseases, could be possible. In bioethical documents, the dividing line is drawn between "health purposes" and "enhancement." Even if this line is continuously redefined, it is still an option for restricting "the benefit of the whole" to a reduction of health burdens.[10] Of course, this could be used to support the view that prospective parents have a general genetic obligation to give birth to the healthiest possible children, as for instance Robert Edwards argues.[11] This naturally also introduces the prevention of disease as a justification for selection (of embryos and fetuses). This implies either that being put to death is better for a human being than having a disease, or that the burden of an ill individual who depends on others is unreasonable. With this in mind, a plausible morality of exceptions in border-line situations easily turns into the moral command that competent individuals should bring about an indirect "benefit of the whole" through their decisions. In addition, interests can be influenced by an appropriate offer, by social expectations, and by the reduction of the dignity argument regarding early human life forms to a piety argument.

How should we assess the eugenics argument under these circumstances? Morally, it can be summed up as an argument against the collectivism of population genetics ("the benefit of the whole") and against the misuse of self-determination at the cost of others ("indirect eugenics"). In the first case, the argument is directed against the preservation of individual human dignity, in the second, against the consideration of the anthropological status of not yet competent human beings or those humans who no longer seem to be competent (the euthanasia problem). Because of this, the eugenics argument is dependent on those parameters which differentiate individual well-being and individual rights from general welfare options. Here, the morality of autonomy (self-determination and self-obligation) is a good antidote. In the case of indirect eugenics, of course, the moral discussion shifts to the moral obligations of protecting embryos. However, I shall not discuss this issue here. Instead I shall turn to another argument which often appears in relation to human genetics, namely the slippery slope argument.

The slippery slope argument

The slippery slope argument has been articulated by Barbara Guckes as follows.[12] Someone might not reject an action A as such but tries to show that by allowing this action other actions will necessarily follow and one of those which appear later in the chain is to be rejected for moral reasons. This means that the moral weighing of action A is burdened with the negative consequences that arise, and the scale is tipped toward the negative.

Objections to the consistency of this argument focus on the claim of inevitability. The action-chain can possibly be interrupted, although from an experiential point of view the inevitability may be a plausible prognosis. The plausiblity of the prognosis, however, is more like a kind of warning of potential consequences than an argument in itself. It is much more likely that a plausible prognosis of consequences based on analogous experiences will solidify an already existing negative inclination.

In relation to human genetics, there are negative prognoses of consequences on the slope of genetic diagnosis (including screening programmes that serve the interests of insurance companies and employers) and on the slope of gene therapy (including germ-line cell therapy and programmes of population genetics). It is claimed that due to the accelerating increase of the number of possibilities caused by scientific and technological progress a strict line can only be defended at the beginning. This argument is not one of logical necessity but of experiential analogy. Of course, the objection remains: with what justification does one stop at one particular point a chain of events which in principle is unending? This argument of infinite regress could nonetheless be made even stronger by the argument that once a chain of events has tipped to the morally negative side of the balance it cannot recover from this downward course. But to this it can be replied that from a historical perspective good has sometimes also been the outcome of the bad.

Thus the slippery slope argument remains a relative argument based on experience. It can play a role in evaluation, but more in the sense of a tutorial with regard to the breaking of taboos. Once the taboos have been broken and the ethical justification has been handed over to other arguments, then the slippery slope argument will no longer be regarded as morally decisive but only as a post-moral motive. Those who worry, for example, about a slippery slope from "health purposes" to "enhancement" base their worries, not without reason, on certain tendencies. However, they can morally reject an action A (for example, somatic gene transfer) only if there are specific ethical reasons for this. Those, however, who find action A to be questionable anyway, for example, because of the selection of anthropologically equal living beings due to the decisions of others, will try to "para-ethically" reinforce this negative assessment by using analogous experiences in order to point out a negative trend. Of course, one must note that the cause of the negative chain of events to which the action A could lead may not actually lie in the action itself, but rather in, for example, scientific curiosity, economic power, or the lack of awareness of the persons requesting the technologies. In the final analysis, we are dealing with justified expectations of possible misuse. Arguments of misuse at the level of empirical prognostication cannot invalidate the moral permissibility of a practice (abusus non tollit usum). But they are, of course, strong additional arguments when an action already appears as an "abusus."

Summary

Rational justification of moral judgements regarding the sensitive and emotionally loaded problems of human genetics is an important requirement if an argumentative discourse in practical ethics is to be possible. Yet there are also arguments that are posed as "moral" which are not, or not primarily, concerned with whether a position, an action, or an institution is right or wrong in the ethical sense. Rather, they are concerned with attitudes to technology, goods, or individual conflicts which either already exist prior to the morally reflective and argued judgement or assume it in advance. Dealing with prejudices prevents them from becoming unexamined prejudices. The illumination of strategic accessories which are meant to strengthen the plausibility of moral judgements is also a part of the clarification of the argumentation. While the boundaries between presuppositions, moral arguments, and strategic efforts are to be analytically differentiated, they nonetheless also intersect each other, since concrete moral judgements always present a "mixtum compositum" of description, judgement, and expectation. This is especially true when a theological context of ethical argumentation is invoked.

Notes

1. Rehmann-Sutter, Müller (eds.), 1995.
2. Cf. Ibid., p. 108.
3. Fuchs, 1996, pp. 135–170.
4. Cf. BAK Guidelines, January 1995, p. 138
5. Sass, 1991.
6. See Habermas, 1994.
7. See Graumann, 1999; Reich (ed.), 1995.
8. See Hirchhorn, Mieth,1969.
9. Horz, 1991.
10. On this, see Haker, 1993.
11. See Edwards, 1998.
12. See Guckes, 1997. See also Paul, 1997.

Bibliography

Bayertz, K., (Hrsg.), 1996. Moralischer Konsens. Technische Eingriffe in die menschliche Fortpflanzung als Modellfall. Suhrkamp: Frankfurt.

Bayertz, K., Schmidtke, J., Schreiber, H.-J., (Hrsg.), 1995. Somatische Gentherapie (Medizinische, ethische und juristische Aspekte. Gustav Fischer: Stuttgart, Jena, NewYork.

Bonss, W., Hohlfeld, R., Kollek, R., 1992. "Risiko und Kontext. Zur Unsicherheit der Gentechnologie." In: Bechmann, G., Rammert, W. (eds.). *Technik und Gesellschaft.* Jahrbuch 6, Frankfurt a.M., pp. 141–174.

Davis, B. D., 1992. "Germ-line therapy: Evolutionary and moral considerations". *Human Gene Therapy* 3, pp. 361–363.

De Wachter, M. A. M., 1993. *Experimental (somatic) gene therapy. Ethical concerns and control.* Maastricht.

Edwards, R. G., 1998. "Introduction and development of IVF and its ethical regulation." In: E. Hildt, E., Mieth, D. (eds.). *In Vitro Fertilisation in the 1990s. Towards a Medical, Social and Ethical Evaluation.* Ashgate: Aldershot, pp. 3–18.

Fuchs, U., 1996. *Gentechnik, Der Griff nach dem Erbgut, Eine kritische Bestandsaufnahme.* Bergisch-Gladbach: Lübbe.

Graumann, S., 1999. *Ethische Probleme der Gentherapie.* Unpublished dissertation, Tübingen.

Guckes, B., 1997. *Das Argument der schiefen Ebene.* Urban und Fischer: München.

Habermas, J., 1994. *Faktizität und Geltung. Beiträge zur Diskurstheorie des Rechts und des demokratischen Rechtsstaates.* Suhrkamp: Frankfurt a. M.

Haker, H., 1993. "Human Genome Analysis and Eugenics". In: Haker, H., Hearn, R., Steigleder, K. (eds.). *Ethics of Human Genome Analysis: European Perspectives.* Francke: Tübingen , pp. 290–323.

Hirchhorn, K., Mieth, D., 1969. "Genetische Manipulation des Menschen." *Wort und Wahrheit* 24, pp. 346–371.

Horz, 1991. "Eugenics." In: *Philos WB der NW.* Berlin.

Müller, S., Simon, J. W., Vesting, J. W., 1997. *Interdisciplinary approaches to gene therapy, legal, ethical and scientific aspects.* Springer-Verlag: Heidelberg, Berlin, New York.

Orkin, S. H., Motulsky, A. D., 1995. *Report and Recommendations of the Panel to Assess the NIH Investment in Research on Gene Therapy.* National Institutes of Health: Bethesda.

Paul, S., 1997. "Genetic Testing: Sliding Down the Slippery Slope?" *Biomedical Ethics, Newsletter of the European Network for Biomedical Ethics* 2, 3, pp. 69–73.

Petermann, T., Schmitt, J. J., 1996. *Monitoring 'Gentherapie'. Die rechtliche Regelung der Gentherapie im Ausland (eine Dokumentation.* TAB-Arbeitsbericht Nr. 40 des Büro für Technikfolgen-Abschätzung beim Deutschen Bundestag. Bonn.

Rehmann-Sutter, C., Müller, H. (Hrsg.). 1995. *Ethik und Gentherapie. Zum praktischen Diskurs um die molekulare Medizin.* Attempto: Tübingen.

Reich, W. (ed.), 1995. "Eugenics." In: *Encyclopedia of Bioethics.* Free Press: New York.

Sass, H.-M., (Hrsg.), 1991. *Genomanalyse und Gentherapie. Ethische Herausforderungen in der Humanmedizin.* Springer Verlag: Berlin, Heidelberg, New York.

Schmitt, J. J., Hennen, L., Petermann, T., 1994. *Stand und Perspektiven naturwissenschaftlicher und medizinischer Problemlösungen bei der Entwicklung gentherapeutischer Heilmethoden.* TAB-Arbeitsbericht Nr. 25 des Büro für Technikfolgen-Abschätzung beim Deutschen Bundestag. Bonn.

Wimmer, R., 1989. "'Kategorische Argumente' gegen die Keimbahn-Gentherapie? Eine Prüfung der Stellungnahme der Enquete-Kommission des Deutschen Bundestages." In: Wils, J.-P., Mieth, D. (ed.). *Ethik ohne Chance? Erkundungen im technologischen Zeitalter.* Attempto: Tübingen, pp. 182–209.

RIHITO KIMURA

Genetic Diagnosis and Gene Therapy in the Cultural Context: Social and Bioethical Implications in Japan

Introduction: genetics and public policy

Issues and problems related to human genetics, and in particular to genetic disease, are attracting much attention in Japan today. The rapid development of genetic science has increased the potential of genetic diagnosis and gene therapy as a means for the treatment of currently incurable diseases such as cancer and AIDS. However, even though there might be no direct threats of ideological manipulation by genetic science at present, we should not forget the numerous and tragic mistakes that have been committed in the name of human welfare and progress throughout the world in conjunction with supposedly "genetic" or "eugenic" legislation.[1] Moreover, we must remember the intentional harm to human genes caused by the Atomic Bombs in Hiroshima and Nagasaki in 1945 and the use of the defoliant "Agent Orange" in Vietnam. I had direct contact with victims of the latter during my stay in Saigon in the beginning of 1970s.[2]

Clearly, science and technology need to be guided by a bioethical public policy. For, as history teaches us, if there is no opportunity for public scrutiny, science and technology are more likely to be used for military and dehumanizing purposes.

This is one of the reasons why ecumenical organizations such as The World Council of Churches have had a series of consultations on science, technology and religion in the face of rapid social change. I had the opportunity of participating in one of the pioneering conferences held in Zurich in 1973 on the issue of "Genetics and the Quality of Life." The participants were theologians, lawyers, policy makers, and medical experts, including Dr. Robert Edwards, the first person to carry out a successful birth of an in vitro fertilized baby, Louise Brown (1978).[3] I still remember the dialogue with eminent physiologists, theologians and ethicists on the necessity for the open and public participation of lay-people in order to lay down bioethical public policies and guidelines for the sound future development of medical and scientific technologies.

In Japan, due to the lack of timely input from traditional religious organizations etc., there is a risk that society will repeat past mistakes in the face of new innovative types of medico-technological applications and scientific developments, in particular with respect to genetic science, including human genome analysis.[4]

Genetic diagnosis of familial cancer in Japan and the proposed Ethical Guidelines of 1998

For many years, the Japanese word "Iden Byo" (genetic disease) has had a rather negative connotation. Some people believe that the appearance of genetic disease in a family member indicates some sort of wrong-doing in the previous generation. This belief is based on a traditional Japanese idea which may originate from the Buddhist notions of Karma or destiny.[5]

Genetic disease was regarded as shameful to the family and something to be hidden and kept secret, in particular because genetic diagnosis and disease might result in social discrimination against a particular "family clan" when it comes to marriage, employment, schooling, etc. One important aspect of genetic disease in Japan is that it is not only a matter for the individual and the immediate family members, but also for the whole generational family.

Ethics of familial cancer research in Japan

Serious bioethical issues are raised by familial cancer diagnosis. Openness among family members is often not the norm in the case of serious disease. Misdirected efforts to cure the patient are made, and false hopes for recovery are proclaimed. In the case of terminal illness, such as cancer, the patient would not be told the truth that he or she is dying. However, if the situation is not terminal, but involving genetic defects or diseases like breast cancer or familial polyposis coli, the individual patient would be told the facts, but he or she would usually not tell the truth to other family members who might be affected by similar genetic defects in the future. This illogical contrast in not telling the truth to the patient in the terminal stage of cancer (not telling the truth to a dying patient) while presenting the genetic diagnosis of familial cancer (but not telling the truth to other family members at risk) might be interpreted as a psychological protection mechanism in Japanese culture. This mechanism aims at preserving a gentle feeling of loving-kindness without telling the "truth" in order to avoid the harmful reality.

However, the traditional ethos of the Japanese people has been changing during the last twenty years, at least slowly.

Patients and the formation of the "Family Support Group"

One example of slow change is the formation of the patient and family self-help group called "Harmony Line."[6] This organization had around 40 members at its establishment in 1998. Two thirds of its members are patients themselves; the rest are relatives. The purpose of this organization is to share and exchange various kinds of information regarding their disease, living conditions, medication, surgery, alternative treatment, etc.[7]

In this social and cultural context, the Ethics Committee of The Japanese Society for Familial Tumor (JSFT) in 1998 presented its draft guidelines for familial cancer research and clinical trial.[8] JSFT was originally formed to be a key research station for Familial Cancer and Prevention Project of UICC (Unio Internationalis Contra Cancrum) in the Asia-Oceania region.[9]

The outline of Genetic Diagnosis Research Guidelines

JSFT's Ethics Committee had been working on these draft cancer research guidelines since 1996. Below follows a brief summary,[10] which I have paraphrased to denote the main elements of each clause in the original Japanese text.[11]

In the Introductory Notes, the guidelines explain the purpose of familial cancer research and other relevant issues, such as the meaning of susceptibility, the protection of privacy, the guarantee of human rights and dignity of patients and family, and the necessity of ethical consideration in order to carry out scientific work.

In addition, the following nineteen recommendations are put forward.

I. Fundamental Principle of the Guidelines.

1. The priority of genetic diagnosis and research in familial cancer should be the protection of the human rights of the concerned participants and family members as it relates to the whole lineage of the family.

II. Purpose and Conditions of Research.

2. The research should only be performed for the advancement of diagnostic, therapeutic and prophylactic procedures, as well as the understanding of the etiology and pathogenesis of disease. Medically non-relevant research should not be performed.

3. Prior to carrying out a genetic test, it is necessary for the participants and society in general to make a comparative medical, psychological and social study of the balance between expected advantages and disadvantages. The test will be carried out when its advantage is confirmed and the informed consent has been obtained from the subjects.

4. The selection of participants should only be based on those individuals who have a probable genetic susceptibility due to various familial and clinical

data. Moreover, in the case of carrying out genetic tests on minors, the tests should be beneficial directly to them.

5. Genetic diagnosis should be performed by a physician who has an understanding of the meaning and limitations of genetic testing.

6. The research should be in accordance with ethical principles expressed in the Helsinki Declaration of the World Medical Association. Justification of the research should be stated clearly and in detail in the protocol.

7. The protocol for research and application of genetic diagnosis in medical services should be reviewed by a proper institutional ethics board.

III. Informed Consent.

8. Prior to genetic diagnosis research and the taking of samples, the participant should be made aware of the following, orally or in writing: the aim, the procedure, the expected benefits, the potential disadvantage (the possibility of having mental stress), the limitations of genetic testing (i.e. the occurrence of false positives or negatives) and the protection of privacy. Moreover, it is necessary for the physician to obtain the consent of the subject based on his or her free will. The consent should be secured in writing.

9. In genetic diagnosis and research, detailed discussions concerning the research should be carried out in order to obtain an informed consent from the participant. The premise is that he or she should be informed about the name and condition of the disease.

10. The participant has a right to refuse genetic sample testing and there should not be any medical disadvantage due to this refusal. Moreover, he or she may also change the decision in due course without receiving any negative outcome.

11. In receiving genetic diagnosis and testing, the participant should be informed clearly that while there might be potential advantages in terms of better treatment and prevention, there are also potential social disadvantages with respect to marriage and conflicts among the lineage family members.

12. The participants should be clearly informed whether particular genetic tests and diagnoses are still on the experimental stage or are established procedures of medical practice. It should be explained that at this stage the majority of genetic diagnoses have been carried out for research purposes.

13. Third parties such as parents, guardians or proxies could be given the right to consent on behalf of non-competent participants if this is in the patient's best interests.

14. The result of the genetic test and diagnosis should be disclosed to the participant, if he or she wants to know, and should be withheld if he or she prefers not to know. The possible benefits and disadvantages of declining information should be explained to the participant.

IV. Maintenance and Protection of the Genetic Information of the Individual.
15. The right to have access to genetic information belongs to the participant. Right to have access to the information could also be possible for medical staff members and researchers.

16. The maintenance and confidentiality of genetic information of the individual should be strictly controlled in order to protect the privacy of the participants.

17. The maintenance of the detailed genetic information of the individual and the registration of the genetic information of the family lineage of the participants is necessary for the advancement of the study of familial cancer and for securing its scientific quality.

V. Support Systems for the Participants.
18. It is necessary to provide genetic counseling in keeping with the need of individuals and family members and in response to their psychological changes.

19. The arrangement of a medical, psychological and social support system in receiving the opinion of the subjects and the support group is recommended.

A break-through for medical research in Japan

As I mentioned above, these guidelines are the result of the continuous efforts by JSFT which began in 1996.[12] We see in them a full recognition of the principle of respect for the autonomy of the participants in research and of the fundamental idea of informed consent in genetic diagnosis, testing and research. After detailed discussions on drafts and amendments, the Ethics Committee finally presented them at a general assembly of JSFT in 1998.[13]

In our cultural context, the ethical aspects of research on the genetic problems of individuals always raise the complicated question of family relationship and conflict. However, I think that these JSFT guidelines reflect a very well refined sensitivity to the family issues as well as the participant-centered, anti-paternalistic research on genetic diagnosis and testing. This is for many Japanese medical researchers a radical departure. And this is one of the reasons why, after three years of repeated revision, presentation and amendment, these guidelines still remain a "proposal" (a draft) without receiving the official endorsement of the general assembly of JSFT.

Ethical aspects of gene therapy and informed consent in Japan

In this section, I shall focus on the recently emerging gene therapy and some bioethical problems of the research protocol including informed consent documents.

Guidelines for gene therapy in Japan

In February 1994, the "Guidelines for Gene Therapy Clinical Research" (GGTCR) were issued as an official "Notice No. 23" of the Ministry of Health and Welfare (MHW) followed by similar guidelines by the Ministry of Education.[14] By this Notice, a review board, the so-called Central Evaluation Committee for Gene Therapy, was established. Some of its members have assigned memberships in committees of both the Ministry of Health and Welfare and the Ministry of Education.

According to these guidelines, genetic manipulation for the enhancement of the body or particular abilities by using germ-cells should be discouraged and even prohibited[15] as is the case in many countries in the world. This is also in line with statements issued by international organizations such as WHO, CIOMS, UNESCO and the Council of Europe.

A 1991 survey carried out by the Prime Minister's Office has shown that more than 50% of the public supports gene therapy.[16] Moreover, professionals argue that the medico-technological intervention on particular genes for the purpose of gene therapy would be justified bioethically and legally if the patient's situation is regarded as incurable, and if the patient agrees to become involved with full informed consent.

I think that in the public debate on gene therapy, contributions from various disciplines such as bioethics, religion, philosophy, genetics and medicine are extremely important and even necessary. Furthermore, open communication between the general public and the experts should be a basic factor in all public policy-making and regulation.[17]

The first gene therapy protocol in Japan was carried out at Hokkaido University Hospital in 1995. The subject was a patient with ADA deficiency. According to a report published in 1997, after 11 rounds of treatment, the patient's condition had improved. This case received quite a lot of attention in the Japanese media as an innovative new medical technology to be applied to very rare types of disease.

Review of scientific and ethical quality

In the spring of 1997, the National Commission on Health and Welfare Policy[18] was officially established at the Ministry of Health and Welfare. Its Subcommittee for the Evaluation of Advanced Technology of Medicine has been functioning as a national review board for gene therapy research since 1997 when it replaced the former Central Evaluation Committee for Gene Therapy.

As a member of this National Commission and its Subcommittee for the Evaluation of Advanced Technology of Medicine,[19] I have been involved in the public review of scientific and ethical aspects of several gene therapy protocol applications.

In 1998, the Subcommittee reviewed applications of gene therapy protocol for kidney cancer at the Hospital of Tokyo University's Medical Research Institute, for lung cancer at the Hospital of Okayama University Medical School, for esophageal cancer at Chiba University Hospital, and for breast cancer at the Cancer Research Society's Hospital in Tokyo.

Common to many of the applications were insensitive and immature phrases used without serious attention to the patient's and family's feelings, and this in spite of the emphasis of the Guidelines on the "protection of patient's rights and respect for human dignity."[20] For example, one research protocol justified its purpose by mentioning that "[t]his experimental gene therapy treatment is not quite verified yet because of lack of data about the cure of disease and because the risk factors are not known in detail. But, this would not be of any obvious harm to a patient who is in the terminal stage of life". This can be intepreted as: "The researcher still does not know the degree of risk or safety of this gene therapy. However, the patient is going to die soon anyway. So this could be justifiable."[21] The patient, the family, and the general public would certainly be much offended by these so-called "scientifically and medically accurate and objective phrases."

According to GGTCR, the subject must be confronted with lethal and fatal sickness such as severe hereditary disease, cancer, AIDS and other life-threatening diseases. Moreover, in Chapter 1, section 2 and 3 it is stated that the expected benefits of this clinical research should be superior to those of presently existing alternative methods, and that the benefit to the patient should outweigh the foreseeable disadvantages.

In accordance with the GGTCR, the insensitive ways of writing research protocols, disregarding the rights and dignity of the patients, should be avoided. This is particularly important in the Japanese cultural context.

A scientifically oriented mind sometimes leads researchers into hasty expectations of positive results in an "If it works, it's O.K." mentality without serious consideration of the fact that the patient places his or her last hope in gene therapy. However, this mentality could also be regarded as a result of a cultural tradition of medical paternalism in Japan.[22]

It is very important to mention here that the GGTCR state their objectives to be both to ensure scientific and ethical validity and to promote the proper conduct of gene therapy clinical research.

The difference between "claim" and "revoke"

In the research protocol documents of various institutions, it is stated that the patient is "able to claim" to stop the experimental procedure anytime he or she wants. This expression might seem quite acceptable to a medical expert. However, as a lawyer-bioethicist, I have pointed out in the committee that there is a problem with the phrase "able to claim" to stop and insisted that this vague statement should be revised. I proposed an amendment which changes this phrase to "the experimental treatment of gene therapy should be definitely halted due to the claim of the patient". Otherwise, I stressed, there would be cases of patients being "able to claim" to stop the experimental treatment but not being able to actually stop it. And, once it has begun, patients and family are usually not "claiming" since there is no guarantee of "halting" the treatment.[23]

The GGTCR state more accurately that any subject who has consented to gene therapy can "revoke" his or her agreement anytime.[24] The difference between "able to claim" and "revoke" is obvious from the patients' point of view.

In addition to the lack of sensitivity expressed in research protocols, Subcommittee members have also recognized the limited number of references to the variety of existing and possible alternative treatments. Moreover, the protocols sometimes lack detailed description of the nature of the disease to which the experimental treatment of gene "therapy" would be applied. Even among medical experts the application of the word "therapy" for this gene transfer is questioned due to the present limited success rate for the cure of disease by this procedure. Particularly in the case of a "clinical research trial of gene therapy", a balanced description of the benefit to patients is vital.

After evaluating several gene therapy protocols, a majority of the Subcommittee members including myself concluded that many of them were not written well enough to be understood by lay-people such as patients and their families. The majority also concluded that sometimes they were written in a manner that was insensitive to the patient's and family's states of mind which are usually characterized by a hope for complete cure.

As mentioned above, there is in Japan a cultural difficulty of having straight communication between patients and physicians with respect to disease. However, in accordance with international trends of research ethics and protocol review process, the Japanese Gene Therapy Guidelines of 1994 state the full assurance of "informed consent." The rapid development of high-technology medicine and its application to the cure of diseases has various implications in our particular cultural, social context. However, we also have to recognize the positive challenge to change traditional values in this particular cultural context, especially in the ethics of medical research.[25]

Concluding remarks: towards patient-centered research

Finally, I shall try to explain these attitudes of Japanese scientists doing research on genetic diagnosis and gene therapy. First, there are remains of a paternalistic medical tradition. It has been difficult for many Japanese to ask questions to superiors and authoritative persons such as physicians, teachers and government bureaucrats.

Second, in Japan there is an "Amae" (sense of dependency) mentality to the superiors and the professionals including parents. This sense of "Amae" is uniquely characterized as one of the components of the Japanese personality which is naturally reflected in the mind of the Japanese patient. According to this interpretation, patients are traditionally expected to be dependant on the physicians, nurses and other medical staff members without asking any questions. They are usually making their decisions in a communal, familial and contextual manner. The decision is usually not based on purely individualistic and autonomous considerations.[26] As a matter of fact, the person with a very independent and individualistic behavior would be regarded as an egocentric person, and might be blamed for lacking the sense of dependency which is the basis for communal living in the Japanese cultural context.

Third, quite a number of Japanese have a feeling of resentment against the arrogant, authoritative professional dominance of medical experts. This could be symbolized in the unhappy memories of the first heart transplants in Japan in 1978, which were a failure and led to accusations of murder against the paternalistic surgeon (although he was not prosecuted).[27]

The lack of openness among professionals, particularly in the field of advanced medical sciences, is a very serious issue, since the public sometimes does not properly understand the application of new medical technology such as organ transplants, genetic engineering, and gene therapy. Therefore, it is good that GGTCR have proposed a more open public review system by gathering experts from different fields such as molecular biology, genetics, clinical pharmacology, pathology, law, and bioethics, and also inviting clinical experts on the particular disease regarding which the gene therapy is to be performed.

To be sure, the attitudes to informed consent are changing.[28] Decision-making becomes more individual and autonomous. However, some traditional family values remain, for instance the practice of not telling the truth to other family members when sharing a common fate such as unexpected disease or terminal disease. But, even though family values and bonding have some positive aspects, I believe that the Japanese should not be encouraged to justify a violation of human dignity and human rights in the name of culture or tradition.

In the process of application of new medical technology, we need to establish an open, public, and internationally acceptable Bioethics Public Policy. In doing so, traditional attitudes, typical for an Asian cultural context, and in particular for Japan, could be seriously challenged.

Within the framework of a bioethical reconceptualization, the study of the Japanese situation regarding genetic diagnosis and gene therapy shows a possibility for changes of the Japanese public policy with respect to the cure of patients suffering from genetic disease.[29]

Regarding these trends of value change in the Japanese culture, it is very important to note that the background document on clinical gene therapy research issued by the Health Science Council in April 1993 is a positive sign of public understanding. It states: "Thus, researchers and related individuals should make efforts to gain the understanding of the general public by always being aware of social and ethical problems, conducting research with these issues in mind, by explaining clearly what gene therapy is, by informing subjects very well in each case of clinical research, by actively making information open to the public, and actively disclosing it to the public."[30]

This is one of the accomplishments of the bioethical input to public policy-making in Japan. Moreover, the Japanese public has also got an opportunity to be present in protocol review sessions, from time to time, which has never been the case before. And all the minutes of the Council meetings, committees and sub-committees are in the public domain and available through the internet homepage of the Ministry of Health and Welfare.[31]

I conclude by stressing once again that a well-informed public and advanced hi-tech medical experts should work together towards achieving the hope of full care and cure of patients with fatal and hopeless diseases.

Notes

1. Kimura, 1991a.
2. Spinsanti, 1995.
3. Abrecht, 1973.
4. Kimura, 1991b.
5. Ohkura, Kimura, 1989.
6. Fellowship Association for the Patients of Polyposis Coli.
7. Gondo, 1998.
8. JSFT, 1998.
9. Utsunomiya, 1998.
10. A revised version, May 30th, 1998.
11. Ethics Committee, JSFT, 1998.
12. Tsunematsu, Kakee, 1998.
13. JSFT, 1998.
14. MHW, 1994.
15. MHW, 1994. Chapters 1–6.
16. Prime Ministers Office, 1991.
17. National Institutes of Health, 1990, pp. 6–7.
18. Kosei Kagaku Shingikai.
19. Sentan Iryo Gijyutsu Hyoka Bukai.
20. NCHW, 1998. Chapter 2, section 3.
21. Tokyo University, 1998.
22. Kimura, 1995.
23. MHW, 1998.
24. MHW, 1994. Chapter 3–5.
25. Kimura, 1995.
26. Doi, 1973.
27. Kimura, 1991 c.

28. Kimura, 1993.
29. Kimura, 1990.
30. Kimura, 1993.
31. URL: http://www.mhw.go.jp.

Bibliography

Abrecht, P. et.al., 1975. *Genetics and Quality of Life*. Pergamon Press: Elmsford, New York.

Doi, T., 1973. *The Anatomy of Dependence*. Kodansha International: Tokyo.

Ethics Committee, JSFT, 1998. "Guidelines for Research in Familial Tumor Diagnosis and its Clinical Application." *Molecular Medicine: Familial Tumor*, Special Issue No. 473 (in Japanese), pp. 376–382.

Gondo, N., et.al., 1998. "Suggestions from Patients Group." *Molecular Medicine: Familial Tumor*, Special Issue No. 473 (in Japanese), pp. 168–170.

Hospital of Medical Research Institute, Tokyo University, Gene Therapy Protocol, 1998 (in Japanese), p. 25.

Kimura, R., 1990. "Religious Aspects of Human Genetic Information." In: Chadwick, D. (ed.). *Human Genetic Information: Science, Law and Ethics*. Ciba Foundation Symposium 149. John Wiley & Sons: New York.

Kimura, R., 1991a. "Jurisprudence in Genetics." In: Blyzhenkov, V. et. al.(eds.). *Ethical Issues of Molecular Genetics in Psychiatry*. Springer-Verlag: Berlin, pp.157–168.

Kimura, R., 1991b. "Das japanische Forschungsprojekt." In: Sass, H.-M. (ed.). *Genomanalyse und Gentherapie*. Springer-Verlag: Berlin, pp.163–170.

Kimura, R., 1991c. "Japan's Dilemma with the Definition of Death." *Kennedy Institute of Ethics Journal* 1, 2, pp. 123–131.

Kimura, R.,1993. "Asian Perspectives: Experimentation on Human Subjects in Japan—Bioethical Perspectives in a Cultural Context." In: Bankowski, Z. et. al. (ed.). *Ethics and Research on Human Subjects: International Guidelines*. Council for International Organizations of Medical Sciences: Geneva, pp. 181–187.

Kimura, R., 1995. "History of Medical Ethics, Contemporary Japan." In: Reich, W. (ed.). *Encyclopedia of Bioethics*. Macmillan: New York, pp. 1496–1505.

Ministry of Health and Welfare, Notice no.23, 1994. *Guidelines for Gene Therapy Clinical Research*. MHW: Tokyo.

National Institutes of Health, 1990. *Governmental Oversight and Public Participation*. Washington DC, pp. 6–7.

Ohkura, K., Kimura, R.,1989. "Ethics and Medical Genetics in Japan." In: Wertz, D. C., Fletcher J.C. (eds.). *Ethics and Human Genetics: A Cross Cultural Perspective*. Springer-Verlag: New York, pp. 294–316.

Spinsanti, S., 1995. *La bioetica*. FrancoAngeli: Milano, pp. 133–139.

Tsunematsu, Y., Kakee, N., 1998. "Clinical and Research Problem." *Molecular Medicine: Familial Tumor*, Special Issue No. 473 (in Japanese), pp. 134–139.

Utsunomiya, J., 1998. "The Concept of Familial Tumor." *Molecular Medicine: Familial Tumor*, Special Issue No. 473 (in Japanese), pp. 11–19.

Testing, Screening, Selecting, Treating, Preventing

KRIS DIERICKX

The Impact of Human Gene Therapy on Genetic Screening and Testing: Ethical and Societal Considerations

Introduction

During the last years, no science seems to be more laden with expectations and questions than medical genetics. In daily life, genes, DNA and heredity are referred to from many different perspectives. In popular culture the DNA has become a sacred entity, a way to explore fundamental questions about human life, to define the essence of human existence, and to imagine immortality.[1] In this huge area of genetics we can distinguish several fields of application. At the moment, gene therapy is getting most attention from the media and the broad public. An application which is much less well known and has received much less attention is the practice of genetic testing and screening. In this article we present some theses on the mutual implications of gene based therapy and genetic screening. First of all, we shall analyse in more detail the meaning of 'gene therapy' and 'genetic screening'.

Gene therapy

The original idea behind gene therapy is to replace defective genes in patients suffering from monogenetic hereditary diseases such as Huntington's disease and cystic fibrosis with genes that function correctly. In the course of time, the term has taken on a broader meaning and it is now, in effect, the general term for any medically motivated transfer of genetic material in humans.[2] This also means that gene transfer methods used in the treatment of, for example cancer are considered to be gene therapy, as are selective alterations in the genetic material of somatic cells as a marking method for diagnosis and scientific research, and the genetic modification of somatic cells for the prevention of disease.[3] We can speak of 'gene therapy' when the intended selective changes are achieved by adding defined genetic material to the cells. Moreover, there must be a modification of the genetic material itself or changes in its transcriptional activity.

Many symptoms can ultimately be traced back to impaired cell function at the molecular level. Detailed knowledge of the mechanisms in question is becoming available for a growing number of genetic affections. This opens up the prospect of intervening at the cellular level for numerous disorders by making specific alterations to the DNA of certain somatic cells. The potential area in which gene therapy can be used is therefore extensive.

We confine our discussion to monogenetic hereditary diseases. Although they are relatively rare, their consequences are usually severe. Despite the progress made during the last years in treating patients with monogenetic affections, many of these disorders lead to an early death. Here gene therapy could offer an opportunity to counterbalance the partial of complete failure of the gene function by inserting 'healthy' genes which could produce the missing protein. This application of gene therapy is *de facto* a form of replacement therapy. This approach would facilitate the definitive removal of the gene cause of the disorder, i.e. the presence of a particalar protein, and make the patient healthy. Examples of monogenetic diseases for which this kind of gene therapy is in being developed, are cystic fibrosis and ADA deficiency.[4]

Genetic screening

Genetic screening is performed within the medical, clinical, and health care context and affects large groups of people. However it receives much less attention than gene therapy. Several authoritative national organs such as the British Nuffield Council on Bioethics, the Dutch Health Council, the French Comité Consultatif d'Ethique and the American Institute of Medicine have published extensive reports on the medical, ethical, social and legal aspects of the implementation of genetic screening programs in general.[5] In addition, international organisations such as the Council of Europe have issued several recommendations and documents concerning this issue,[6] and in different Western countries pilot projects or complete genetic screening programs have been set up.[7]

In the literature there is a whole series of descriptions and definitions of what genetic screening is. For the President's Commission "in a genetic screening an asymptomatic population is tested to identify people who may possess a particular genotype."[8] We define genetic screening as "any kind of test performed for the systematic early detection or exclusion of a hereditary disease or a predisposition to such a disease, or in order to determine whether a person carries a predisposition which may produce a hereditary disease in offspring."[9]

In this definition, three distinctive traits can be distinguished: (1) it concerns an genetic disease, disposition or carriership; (2) there is no reason for the people concerned to look for help; and (3) there is a systematic approach of the target group. In terms of disease and health, a genetic screening program may have the following aims. First, to trace persons with a gene or chromosome composition which may result in, or predispose the persons concerned, to develop a disease. Second, to trace persons with a gene or chromosome composition which may result in, or predispose the descendants of the persons concerned, to develop a disease. Third, to illuminate the frequency of a given genetic disease, a specific disposition, a specific chromosomal rearrangement or possibly a specific combination of genes in the population.[10]

Genetic screening differs from a non-genetic medical screening in at least the following ways.[11] Whereas in both types of screening, identification of persons at risk may lead to the identification of others at risk, in the case of ordinary health screening the connection between persons at risk is often physical proximity (contact), whereas for genetic screening it is by genetic proximity (kinship). Whereas in other forms of health screening the concern is about the subject being screened, in genetic screening the concern is often about the subject's offspring. Third, genetic screening carries an inherent risk of impairing self-image and perceived suitability as a marriage partner or parent.

The applicability of these three characteristics however, can vary with different types of genetic screening. There are three principal types of genetic screening. First, in neonatal screening one seeks genetic mutations in newborn children. It identifies serious genetic diseases at birth, permitting prompt treatment to prevent mental or physical retardation. Phenylketonuria (PKU) was the first condition for which newborn screening was widely adopted. Second, in foetal (prenatal) screening one seeks the disease in the foetus. Foetal screening and prenatal diagnosis identify genetic diseases in the foetus permitting selective termination of pregnancy or the opportunity to prepare the parents for a child with a genetic condition. The most common of these is screening for Down's Syndrome. A third category of genetic screenings is a carrier screening: it identifies individuals heterozygous for a gene for a serious recessive disease that may be at risk for affected offspring. With a prospective genetic carrier screening, individuals and couples can be informed before the birth of the first child about their risk on a child with a genetic affection. The most cited example here is a genetic screening program for carriers of cystic fibrosis, the most common serious autosomal recessive disease in Western society: about one in 25 white persons is a carrier of cystic fibrosis.

Today, the number of genetic mutations, responsible for monogenetic diseases that can be detected by a genetic test is increasing rapidly. One of the main problems with genetic testing in general, and genetic screening in particular, is that once the mutation has been identified, an adequate treatment is possible only in rare cases. For many genetic disorders today, the availability of the genetic test result is not the start of an intensive treatment and curing process. Unfortunately, for many tests for monogenetic disorders, informing people about their genetic status and how to cope with it in order to prevent self-stigmatisation or social discrimination is today the end point. The so-called therapeutic gap leads for certain forms of screening to a new paradigm. Phenotype prevention as an aim for carrier screening for instance is different from the conventional goal of screening and prevention in so far it contains no preventive principle. Instead, generating information to help people coming to an informed decision is considered as an end in itself. This involves a clear change of paradigm for the classic screening philosophy.[12] Confronted with genetics and genetic screening, the classic model of public health seems not to work, because of the actual unchangeability of the human genome.

Genetic screening and the availability of rational gene based therapy: mutual implications

Research into the feasibility of human gene therapy fully explores the practicality and safety of the method on the basis of theoretical understanding and data from animal experiments. In 1980 Mercola and Cline made a first attempt to use gene therapy in patients with beta-thalassaemia, a hereditary disease that affects red blood cells.[13] The trial was broken off prematurely because it had started without any prior ethical assessment and because the protocol was thought to be premature for scientific reasons. In 1989 researchers of the National Institutes of Health (NIH) in the United States finally put forward a research protocol that has gone down in history as the first approved gene therapy in humans. Today more than 350 research protocols with more than 2600 patients have been approved and scientists are convinced that the big breakthrough cannot be far away.

The availability of gene therapy in the (near) future might have a far reaching influence on the medical practice of genetic testing and screening. In this paragraph we will focus on some of the most important possible implications of gene therapy for genetic screening and testing.

Genetic screening can be considered as an obstacle for the development of a rational gene based therapy

Some people argue that for genetic screening programs that are implemented before the development of an adequate human gene therapy for a particular disorder, the screening program might be seen as a well functioning alternative. The resources spent on the realisation and continuation of the genetic screening initiative however, are no longer available for funding research in gene therapy for that particular disease. This becomes clear in a screening program that is considered as one of the most successful, namely the carrier screening for Tay-Sachs. Tay-Sachs disease is a hereditary disorder that occurs primarily, but not exclusively, in Ashkenazi Jewish families from Eastern Europe. The disease is invariably fatal at an early age due to the accumulation of lipid in all body organs.[14] An important purpose of Tay-Sachs screening is to provide eligible clients with genetic counselling about reproductive and mating options. If the purpose, however, is to introduce couples at risk to the benefits of prenatal diagnosis by amniocentesis with the specific intent of recommending abortion of affected foetuses, then screening is not acceptable for orthodox Jews.[15] This last group is concerned about the financial resources consumed by the prenatal genetic screening for Tay-Sachs, because they are afraid that this expense will be a cause that not enough money will be spent to human therapy research for this disorder.

Rational gene based therapy will also sharpen other requirements for a genetic screening program, not only the 'therapy' criterion

Most of the mentioned authoritative reports on genetic screening and testing conclude with a list of requirements for the implementation of a genetic screening program. The most important of these criteria are:[16]

- a direct, simple, sensitive and reliable test method
- informed (education) and free (no external pressure of family, employer, etc) consent
- respect for informational privacy and confidentiality, including the right not to know
- a positive attitude on the part of the target group: the test should be acceptable to affected individuals as well as those to be screened
- facilities for treatment and therapy should be available or early knowledge should be helpful in other ways.

At this moment many are concerned with the last condition. It is now perhaps the key-criterion to be fulfilled, before we start reflecting about the other criteria. For many of those responsible for healthcare, it is the factual obstacle that hinders the implementation of a genetic screening program. Once gene based therapy is available, genetic screening programs are no longer hypothetical thought experiments, but will be implemented in public health care. At present it is also clear that the other criteria are perhaps not just secondary problems in comparison with the availability of an adequate therapy, but might also raise fundamental questions. One example are the formal pleas in the reports on genetic screening in favour of a free consent as a condition for participating in a genetic screening program. Despite the general and fundamental defence of the free consent, the realisation of this criterion for the implementation of a genetic screening program in face of the availability of a rational gene based therapy will no longer be self-evident.[17] In addition to the question to what extent an unrequested screening program can be free, the pressure of health care authorities and insurance companies in order to participate in a genetic screening program that can identify genetic disorders for which there is a human gene therapy will increase. What will be the value of free consent in that context?

For some diseases, rational gene based therapy will be considered to be the only missing factor for the implementation of a genetic screening program

Besides the considerations in our previous thesis, it is clear that in some cases the availability of gene therapy will eliminate the doubts and unclarified questions that are mentioned for other genetic screening programs. If we look to the neonatal PKU screening we see that it is a rather expensive program. There are not so many persons with that disease and in many places obtaining informed consent is neglected. Nevertheless, most specialists agree that it is a good screening program because there is a good treatment program and in Western countries more that 95% of the neonates are screened for it.[18] It is clear that if we are able to offer treatment we will try to identify all persons with the disease in question. The number of genetic screening programs will increase, because one of the main conditions for genetic screening is respected.

The availability of a gene based therapy may lead to a large number of genetic screening programs, but is it always a sufficient reason for implementing genetic screening programs? Furthermore, which genetic modifications are to be called gene therapy? The concepts of health and disease, and of a human person form part of the discussion. What is health? When are we called genetically ill? Do we need a gene therapy?[19] These questions involve the fundamental orientation of medicine. Does medicine regard itself ultimately as a helping and caring profession or as a service institution or an instrument in the hands of administrators responsible for public health and policy?

The impact of the genetic factor will increase. Telling stories about illness and health in the language of genetics, packaging disorders with a genetic label, is of more than literary interest. These narratives might determine the ways problems will be defined, viewed and managed. The stories have consequences for both research and social strategies.[20] Genetics becomes more and more the way to reveal and explain diseases and health. This opens the way to an ongoing process by which differences between individuals are reduced to their DNA codes, with most disorders, behaviours and physiological variations defined (at least in part) as genetic in origin.

From this perspective it is clear that in the light of the availability of rational gene based therapy the importance of the aim of genetic screenings becomes very important. Is the ultimate concern the improvement of the (reproductive) health of individuals or do we focus on the genetic well-being of the group. With the eugenic movement in mind, it is clear that the collective idea of well-being as an aim for social and health care actions does not enjoy a good reputation.[21]

Conclusion

Recent decades have seen impressive advances in our knowledge and understanding of molecular biology. In this article we have focussed on two main developments in this field, namely human gene therapy and genetic screening. Genetic screening programs can already identify people with genetic mutations. Knowledge about gene therapy opens prospects for treating people in the near future with disorders caused by genetic defects. Our study shows that the latter is more than a simple answer to certain needs of the former. The co-existence of the two gene based tools will be not without problems. Moreover, the combination of genetic screening and gene therapy will increase the prospective moral responsibility of individuals and society.

Notes

1. Nelkin, Lindee , 1995, p. 40.
2. Dutch Health Council, 1997, p. 18.
3. Torres, JM, 1995, p. 134.
4. XXX, 1996, p. 1258; Ross, G. *et al.*, 1996, p. 1787.
5. Nuffield Council on Bioethics, 1993; Health Council, 1989 & 1994; Comité Consultatif National d'Ethique, 1995; Institute of Medicine, 1994; Danish Council of Ethics, 1993.
6. Council of Europe, 1990, 1992 & 1994.
7. Hoedemaekers, 1998; Kaback, 1982.
8. President's Commission, p. 2.
9. Health Council, 1994, p. 33.
10. Danish council, 1993, p. 56
11. Rowley, 1984, p. 138.
12. Dierickx, 1997, p. 69.
13. Health Council, 1997, p. 26.
14. Kaback, 1982, p. 244.
15. Rossner, 1991, p. 252.
16. The best known and most cited list of criteria for a screening program is a list of the W. H. O.:
    (1) the condition sought should constitute an important health problem;
    (2) there should be an accepted treatment for patients with recognized disease;
    (3) facilities for diagnosis and treatment should be available;
    (4) there should be a recognizable latent or early symptomatic stage
    (5) there should be a suitable test or examination
    (6) the test should be acceptable to the population
    (7) the natural history of the condition, including development from latent to declared disease, should be adequately understood
    (8) there should be an agreed policy on whom to treat as patients
    (9) the cost of case-finding should be economically balanced in relation to possible expenditure on medical care as a whole
    (10) case-finding should be a continuing process and not a 'once and for all' project
    Wilson & Jungner, 1968, p. 26.

17. Green, & Capron, 1982, p. 496.
18. Verkerk, 1995, p. 2302.
19. Caplan, 1992, p. 128.
20. Lippman, 1992, p. 1470.
21. Juengst, E., 1995, p. 1603.

Bibliography

Caplan, A., 1992. "If gene therapy is the cure, what is the disease?" In: Elias, S., Annas, G. (ed.). *Gene mapping: using law and ethics as guide.* Oxford University Press: New York, pp. 128–142.

Comité Consultatif National d'Ethique pour les Sciences de la Vie et de la Santé, 1995. *Génétique et médecine: de la prédiction à la prévention.* Avis. Rapports: Paris.

Council of Europe, 1990. *Prenatal genetic screening, prenatal genetic diagnosis and associated genetic counselling.* No. R (92). Publishing and Documentation Service: Strasbourg.

Council of Europe, 1992. *Recommendation on genetic testing and screening for health care purposes.* No. R (92) 3. Publishing and Documentation Service: Strasbourg.

Council of Europe, 1994. *Screening as a tool of preventive medicine.* No. R (94) 11. Publishing and Documentation Service: Strasbourg.

Danish Council of Ethics, 1993. *Ethics and mapping of the human genome.* Copenhagen.

Dierickx, K., 1997. "Prevention and predictive genetic health care." In: Anonymous. *Preventive healthcare.* Kluwer Editorial: Diegem, pp. 64–73.

Green, H. P., Capron, A. M., 1982. "Issues of public policy in compulsory genetic screening." In: Beauchamp, T. L.,Walters, L. (eds.). *Contemporary issues in bioethics.* Wadsworth Pub.Co.: Belmont CAL, pp. 494–499.

Health Council of the Netherlands, 1989. *Heredity: science and society. On the possibilities and limits of genetic testing and gene therapy.* Publication nr 31. The Hague.

Health Council of the Netherlands, 1994. *Genetic screening.* Publication nr 22. Den Haag.

Health Council of The Netherlands, 1997. *Gene therapy.* Publication nr 12E. Den Haag.

Hoedemaekers, R., ten Have, H., 1998. "Geneticization: the Cyprus paradigm." *Journal of medicine and philosophy* 23, pp. 274–287.

Institute of Medicine, 1994. *Assessing genetic risks. Implications for health and social policy,* National Academy Press: Washington D.C.

Juengst, E. T., 1995. "'Prevention' and the goals of genetic medicine." *Human gene therapy* 6, pp. 1595–1605.

Kaback, M. M., 1982. "The control of genetic disease by carrier screening and antenatal diagnosis: social, ethical, and medicolegal issues." In: *Birth defects: original article series* 18, 7, pp. 243–254.

Lippman, A., 1992. "Led (astray) by genetic maps: the cartography of the human genome and health care." *Social sciences and medicine* 35, pp. 1469–1476.

Nelkin, D., Lindee, M. S., 1995. *The DNA mystique. The gene as a cultural icon.* W. H. Freeman and Co.: New York.

Nuffield Council on Bioethics, 1993. *Genetic screening. Ethical issues.* London.

President's Commission for the Study of Ethical Problems in Medicine and Biomedical and Behavioral Research, 1983. *Screening and counseling for genetic conditions. A report on the Ethical, Social, and Legal Implications of Genetic Screening, Counseling, and Education Programs*. Washington.

Ross, G., Erickson, R., Knorr, D., et al., 1996. "Gene therapy in the United States: a five-year status report." *Human gene therapy* 7, pp.1781–1790.

Rossner, F., 1991. "Screening for Tay-Sachs disease: a note of caution." *Journal of clinical ethics* 2, pp. 251–252.

Rowley, P. T., 1984. "Genetic screening: marvel or menace?" *Science* 225, pp. 138–144.

Torres, J. M., 1995. "The importance of accurate terminology in the field of human gene transfer." *Human gene therapy* 6, pp. 133–135.

Verkerk, P. H., 1995. "Twintig jaar landelijke screening op fenylketonurie in Nederland" ["Twenty years of nationwide screening for phenylketonuria in the Netherlands"]. *Nederlands tijjdschrift voor geneeskunde [Dutch journal of medicine]* 139, pp. 2302–2305.

Wilson, J. M. G., Jungner, G., 1968. *Principles and practice of screening for disease*. World Health Organization: Geneva.

XXX, 1996. "Human gene therapy clinical trials in Europé." *Human gene therapy* 7, pp. 1258–1259.

NIKOLAUS KNOEPFFLER

Ethical Evaluation of Different Levels of Gene Therapy

When you are in a foreign country, hungry, thirsty and not able to prepare a meal for yourself, you may enter a restaurant. Your fundamental assumption should be that they won't offer you a poisoned meal. If you do not know the names of the different dishes on the menu you may call a waitress. She will explain to you what the names stand for. She will tell you what kind of main course fits with what kind of starter and wine. She may say: "This is our special main course, which I whole-heartedly can recommend." But she should not urge you to take a certain set meal. This decision is up to you.

If you have to make a decision about the moral desirability of embarking on gene therapy, as a physician you may enter an ethical discussion where you sometimes do not know the different ethical concepts. If you ask an ethicist, your fundamental assumption should be that he or she will not offer you an irresponsible ethical approach. The ethicist can explain to you the different ethical concepts and tell you what kind of ethics fits with what kind of decisions. But he or she should not urge you to take a certain decision. This decision is up to you.

Of course, there is an important difference in this comparison with the foreign restaurant: regarding eating and drinking we often apply the latin proverb "de gustibus non disputandum", even if we are astonished if someone orders a burger together with an excellent red wine from the vineyards of Rothschild. In ethics this is not true: we have to dispute because the aim of an ethical discourse is to reach a dialogue between rationalities of the acting persons involved by a mutual disclosure of their motivations, visions and principles. We have to show an openness for new results and should try to find decisions within an open dialogue among all the parties, decisions based on criteria which may be common grounds.

I would like to give you an ethical evaluation of different levels of gene therapeutic interventions in order to prompt kind of discussion. My presentation is based on a study by five members of this Technology-Theology-Sciences Institute in Munich. One of the authors, Ernst-Ludwig Winnacker, is the

President of the Deutsche Forschungsgemeinschaft.[1] I am especially grateful to Prof. Albrecht Sippel, a geneticist from Freiburg[2] with whom I could discuss some of the main points of my paper.

The general approach

I presuppose that human dignity is *the* fundamental principle for any bioethical consensus. The meaning of this principle is best explained by Immanuel Kant's prohibition against completely instrumentalizing human beings.[3] Human beings have an absolute inner value, a dignity. Therefore they are ends in themselves and their interests and welfare must prevail over the sole interest of society or science.

The principle of human dignity is compatible with the medical ethos which aims at improving the health of human beings and at treating human diseases. The principle of human dignity guarantees the autonomy of patients and avoids the use of patients as merely a means for other purposes. The criterion of autonomy implies that the physician discloses to the patient what he wants to do and why. The patient is involved in decision-making. The principle of human dignity guarantees not only the autonomy of the patient directly involved (or the legal representative of a patient not able to consent) but also of the members of society at large. Especially in a field like gene therapy, where new techniques create not only hopes but, at the same time, fears, it is necessary that scientific research is publicly disclosed and discussed.

To summarize: I claim that the principle of human dignity is the fundamental principle of any bioethical consensus. The principle of human dignity implies the medical ethos and the criterion of autonomy in the narrow sense (the patient) and in a broader sense (the members of society).

Four different kinds of genetic interventions and three different levels of therapeutic interventions

I would like to divide genetic engineering into four different kinds of genetic interventions:

1) treatment of diseases
2) prevention of diseases
3) prevention of abnormalities
4) enhancement

But we face problems with this kind of distinction:[4] For example, under the roughly 4000 registered heritable diseases some are by charakter more a handicap than a disease. Take the case of dwarfism. The members of the Society of Little People of America are strictly against any genetical engineering for the purpose of making them taller. It is for them not a therapy, but terror of a genetic norm. On the other hand, there are drugs available, made by recombinant-DNA technology, for treatment of abnormally small people. These drugs are also used by people who wish to be taller even if they are not abnormally small. That means that we face a case of enhancement not of therapy. So the borders between these kinds of interventions are not strict. It is an important task to clarify the concepts of disease and therapy in order to help distinguish between these different levels. We confronted with the ethical question whether enhancement is desirable or not, for example, and with the question of eugenics.

I do not want to deal with these kinds of questions here. Instead, I shall try to evaluate genetic treatment of diseases, commonly called gene therapy, which may include the prevention of heriditary diseases. For that purpose I define three different levels of therapeutic interventions according to their depths of intervention:

1) substitution therapy by drugs produced by gene technology,
2) somatic gene therapy,
3) germ-line gene therapy.

Let us take a closer look at the different levels.

Substitution therapy by drugs produced by gene technology

The first level comprises substitution therapy by drugs produced by means of gene technology. This kind of therapy is morally acceptable as are therapies with drugs not produced by means of gene technology. As soon as the benefits are acknowledged, the risks are known and found acceptable and these drugs are approved of, there is no greater ethical problem than with drugs not produced by gene technology.

Somatic gene therapy

Somatic gene therapy is the second level. Somatic gene therapy is a deeper intervention than therapy using drugs produced by means of gene technology because it is the aim of this intervention to change somatic cells of a patient irreversibly. Nevertheless, this kind of gene therapy is morally unproblematic and is even suggested if there is informed consent, if the treatment is approved of by the responsible medical committees and if the risk-benefit analysis is positive.

Somatic gene therapy normally is not too risky. There is the possibility of a casual integration of transfected DNA which may destroy a coding sequence. If an oncogene is involved this may initiate a transformation of the respective cell. But the relative risk remains between 1 and 25. If the risk to get a certain type of tumor is 1:100000 in that case the risk is at most 25:100000.[5]

Therefore, somatic gene therapy corresponds with the criterion mentioned above, namely the professional medical ethos. Especially in the case of cancer treatment this kind of therapy may improve the survival chances of many patients. But here we face an ethical problem. Normally, the treatment of these kinds of diseases is undertaken, when the patient is near death. The chances of survival are, therefore, very small. On the other hand, there is no real risk of harm to the patient. I would suggest treating patients earlier in time if they have given informed consent after the risks have been explained and understood.

Another ethical problem is as follows: somatic gene therapy may be done on unborn human beings. In the US there are experiments already being done on animal embryos to see whether such kind of therapy could possibly succeed. The aim is to do the same on unborn humans. The US National Institutes of Health started a discussion about the desirability of embarking on *in utero* gene therapy. Critics argue that this move threatens to open up a "slippery slope to eugenics"[6] because the risk of a switch into germ-line gene therapy is high. As long as somatic gene therapy on unborn humans avoids this risk, we can apply the criteria mentioned for the somatic gene therapy on adult patients. If this risk is real, we have to take the ethical evaluation of germ-line therapy into consideration.

Germ-line gene therapy

From the scientific point of view, the intervention by germ-line therapy reaches a new level: This therapy does not only involve the patients themselves, but also their descendants. Germ-line therapy is morally problematic. As you may know, the German law on the protection of embryos, issued after years of fervent discussion, prohibits all research which destroys human embryos. There is again a similar discussion generated by the *Convention on Human Rights and Biomedicine* of the Council of Europe which seems to allow research on embryos until the embryo is fourteen days old although it prohibits germ-line therapy (cf. Art. 13). I do not want to discuss in detail whether a human embryo should be protected from the beginning.[7] But I would like to mention that we have at least three different options:

1) to protect the embryo from the beginning;
2) to protect the embryo after individuation, i. e. after the separation of the embryoblast and trophoblast and when there is no possibility of twins;
3) to protect the embryo after that date, e. g. when the nerve cells develop to a certain stage.

If you think that the embryo should be protected from the beginning, you cannot accept germ-line therapy as long as germ-line therapy destroys embryos for research and needs preimplantation diagnosis—and this will be the case for a very long time to come.

If you do not think so, you will not need to bother with the question of the moral status of the embryo regarding germ-line therapy. A different criteria applies: risk-benefit analysis. Applying the professional medical ethos, you have to choose the treatment which is more reliable, which has fewer risks, better chances and fewer costs. Germ-line therapy is very unreliable. Even after years of research on mice there is only a 10% rate of success.[8] If you apply this kind of technology on humans, you would need preimplantation genetic diagnosis to find out if the therapy has worked. But even if it has worked, you will not know whether there will be a change in the whole system which may prompt malfunctions years after birth.

On the other hand, you can reach the goal of freeing embryos of specified hereditary diseases by preimplantation diagnosis alone in the absence of germ-line therapy. You could implant only the healthy embryos—the same as you would do with embryos after germ-line therapy.

There is only one case in which germ-line therapy alone would work: both parents have the same hereditary disease and the four genes (in the case of recessive diseases) or at least two genes (in the case of dominant diseases) are equally mutated. In these cases only germ-line gene therapy can prevent a hereditary disease. The question is: Do these rare cases, less than 1 couple in 100000,[9] allow us to cross the border between somatic gene therapy and germ-line gene therapy which includes many risks that cannot be calculated?

On March 20, 1998, James Watson, one of the discoverers of the structure of DNA in 1953, and other participants at a symposium organized at the University of California, Los Angeles, asked that no state or federal legislation regulating germ-line gene therapy be passed at that time and that the United States resist any effort by UNESCO or other international bodies to block the exploration of human germ-line engineering.[10]

Ann McLaren critizes Watson's remark "scientists should proceed unhindered towards germ-line engineering." "Either [Watson] has forgotten that the simpler and safer technique of preimplantation genetic diagnosis, already in clinical use, renders germ-line gene therapy for genetic diseases virtually pointless, or it is germ-line engineering for genetic enhancement towards which he wishes to proceed unhindered."[11] Indeed Watson argues for enhancement,[12] if equality is possible, i.e., if every human being has the opportunity to share in this kind of progress. As I told you at the beginning I am not discussing the question as to whether germ-line therapy for other than therapeutical purposes may be morally acceptable or not. But I at least wish to mention one important point worth considering: if we allow germ-line engineering for enhancement we make human beings according to our visions. We have no common grounds here as to what kind of enhancement is desirable or not. It seems, therefore, that we would advance towards instrumentalizing human beings, rather than respecting their being ends in themselves.

This rejection of germ-line engineering for enhancement should not be confused with a further argument against germ-line therapy, the slippery slope argument. It goes as follows: if you accept germ-line therapy to prevent hereditary diseases, you start on the trail towards germ-line engineering. Therefore, you should not embark on this trail at all. I think that slippery slope arguments are bad arguments, because you can abuse everything.[13] You can use a knife to cut a bread and you can use it to kill a person. That does not mean that we should outlaw knives. Therefore, instead of using the slippery slope argument, we should draw the line, where we have good reasons to do this.

I suggest drawing the line between somatic gene therapy and germ-line gene therapy for the reasons given, but I would like to make one important reservation. A supporter of germ-line therapy may object that germ-line therapy and preimplantation genetic diagnosis are not the same. The purpose of germ-line therapy, at most in principle, is to heal a genetic disorder of an embryo and to prevent its descendants from inheriting this disorder. Preimplantation genetic diagnosis instead is not therapy but a way to find out whether the embryo is genetically normal or abnormal. From that, it follows that preimplantation genetic diagnosis implies that you do not have a therapeutic purpose for the genetically abnormal embryo: this embryo won't be implanted. If germ-line therapy worked properly it would be possible to correct the genetic disorder without discarding genetically abnormal embryos. It follows that the rejection of germ-line therapy for the reasons given does not result in a rejection of germ-line therapy in principle.

Conclusion

I would like to summarize my presentation in this table.

Level	Kind of therapy	Ethical evaluation
1st level	Substitution therapy by drugs produced by gene technology	To be viewed like normal drugs
2nd level	Somatic gene therapy	Morally unproblematic, if there is informed consent and the risk-benefit analysis is positive
3rd level	Germ-line therapy to prevent hereditary diseases	Morally unacceptable, because there is a better alternative, PGD (fewer risks, fewer costs) to reach the aim to prevent hereditary diseases

Notes

1. Cf. Winnacker u. a., 1998.
2. Cf. Sippel, 1996.
3. Kant, 1968 (1785), p. 428.
4. Cf. Sippel, 1996, Mouron, Rehmann-Sutter, 1995, Honnefelder 1998, p. 105.
5. Cf. Lindemann, Mertelsmann, 1998, p. 100.
6. *Nature*, Vol. 395, p. 420.
7. Cf. Knoepffler, 1999.
8. Winnacker u. a., 1997.
9. Lindemann, Mertelsmann, 1998, p. 100.
10. Cf. Stock, G., Campbell, J., 1998. *Summary Report: Engineering the Human Germline Symposium*. URL: www.ess.ucla.edu:80/huge/
11. McLaren, 1998.
12. Cf. Watson, 1993.
13. Cf. Beyleveld, 1997, Williams, 1995.

Bibliography

Beyleveld, D., 1997. "The trouble with tendential slippery slope arguments." *Biomedical Ethics* 2, p. 42.

Honnefelder, L., 1998. "Gentherapie. Ethisch." In: Korff, W., Beck, L., Mikat, P. (eds.). *Lexikon der Bioethik*. Gütersloher Verlagshaus: Gütersloh, pp. 104–107.

Kant, I., 1968 (1785). *Grundlegung zur Metaphysik der Sitten*. De Gruyter: Berlin.

Knoepffler, N., 1999. *Forschung an menschlichen Embryonen. Was ist verantwortbar?* Hirzel Verlag: Stuttgart.

Lindemann, A., Mertelsmann R., 1998. "Gentherapie. Problemstand." In: Korff, W., Beck, L., Mikat, P. (eds.). *Lexikon der Bioethik*. Gütersloher Verlagshaus: Gütersloh, pp. 97–102.

McLaren, A., 1998. "Problems of germline therapy." *Nature* 392, p. 645.

Mouron, A., Rehmann-Sutter, C., 1995. "Gentherapie: Ein Katalog offener ethischer Fragen." In: Rehmann-Sutter C., Müller H. (eds.), *Ethik und Gentherapie. Zum praktischen Diskurs um die molekulare Medizin.* Atempto: Tübingen, pp. 22–33.

Sippel, E., 1996. "Gene Therapy—A New Medical Technique and Points to Consider." In: *Jahrbuch für Recht und Ethik 4*, pp. 35–47.

Watson, J., 1993. *Focus* 17, p. 96.

Williams, B., 1995. "Which slopes are slippery?" In: Williams, B., *Making sense of humanity and other philosophical papers.* Cambridge University Press: Cambridge, pp. 213–223.

Winnacker u. a., 1997. *Gentechnik: Eingriffe am Menschen. Ein Eskalationsmodell zur ethischen Bewertung* (2. Aufl.). Herbert Utz: München.

CHRISTIAN MUNTHE

Genetic Treatment and Preselection: Ethical Differences and Similarities

Introduction

The rapid current development in medical genetics and bioscience brings many future prospects for attacking hitherto unresolvable genetic health-problems. However, at least at first glance, these prospects are rather different. In some cases, they relate to actual *treatment* of genetic diseases. In other cases, however, they rather mean *preselecting* individuals free of some genetic defect.

This paper will focus on the ethically relevant differences and similarities between these different ways of approaching genetic disorders. After having described the different strategies which may be used against genetic diseases, I shall discuss to what extent different ethical arguments for and against such interventions place any of the strategies in a more (or less) favourable light. One important conclusion will be that, contrary to what is often assumed, so-called *germ-line* gene therapy is ethically not very different from preselective genetic interventions actually clinically applied today.

Types of genetic interventions in medicine

Treatment of genetic diseases may be of two types: either the gene-product giving rise to the pathological symptoms is manipulated (through drugs, surgery or life-style changes, for instance), or the genetic make-up giving rise to this gene-product is manipulated in such a way that pathological symptoms do not appear. Although the first type of treatment may be highly informed by genetic knowledge, in this paper, I shall focus on the latter type, commonly called gene therapy (GT, for short). I shall also ignore problems involved in making a distinction between pathology and normality, thereby side-stepping the issue of how to distinguish between gene therapy and genetic "enhancement." I shall, however, below question the *desirability* of basing health care policy on such a distinction.

Gene therapy

Although not a present reality, the long-term hope is that GT will eventually enable the reliable, precise and safe *reparation* of specific genetic anomalies. The *ideal* GT thus means that the genome of an individual is modified so as not to give rise to pathological symptoms it would otherwise have given rise to, without any harmful side-effects.[1] Since anyone would agree that *un*reliable, *un*specific and/or *un*safe methods are ethically problematic, I shall assume for the sake of discussion that the ideal GT is already here and consider what could be said for and against it on this assumption.

GT in this sense may be achieved in two ways which are commonly sharply distinguished. First, some of the patient's *somatic* cells may be genetically modified (somatic GT, or S-GT, for short). Such genetic changes will always be "local" in the sense that they will only affect the particular type of cell-line tampered with (for example, skin-cells), and will not be inheritable. Secondly, the patient's *germ-line* cells (early embryonic cells or gametes) may be genetically modified (germ-line GT, or GL-GT, for short). Such changes will affect all types of cells in an individual arising out of such cells, and will also be inheritable.[2]

Genetic preselection

In contrast to GT, *preselective* interventions (GP) do not involve any reparation of a malfunctioning genome. Rather, in this case, genetic information is used as a basis for preventing the occurrence of a possible future individual, who would have had such a genome, to the benefit of *another* possible future individual lacking this genetic anomaly. This result may be achieved in various ways. Perhaps most well-known are prenatal diagnosis and possible selective abortion. However, since this particular method actualises special concerns and controversies,[3] I shall focus on methods proceeding before any pregnancy has been established.

One such method is, of course, the choice of partner when planning to have children. In most cases, this choice is not informed by genetic information but will nevertheless affect *which* children that actually come to exist in the future as well as their genetic make-up. However, in some historic/ethnic/religious settings genetic information obtained from family chronicles has actually been used to settle whether a marriage-licence should be ensued, the most well-known case being Azkenasi Jews, where a serious genetic disease called Tay-Sachs is comparably common. Modern technology offers more sophisticated means that are possible to use also in settings where we do not let our mating be controlled by central authorities, for example (voluntary) genetic testing of possible mating-partners to ensure that there is no risk for the offspring to inherit some disease or disorder.

Most of us would not like to let our choice of partner be guided by such considerations, however.[4] In that case, the medical field of assisted procreation can help with artificial insemination or in vitro fertilisation (IVF) using *donor-gametes*, where the donors have been subjected to genetic testing.[5]

A third method is preimplantation or preconception genetic diagnosis (PGD). These brand new procedures, recently developed within reproductive medicine, enable genetic testing and selection of early embryos (after IVF, but before transfer of any embryo into the uterus of a woman) and, to some extent, of gametes (followed by IVF).[6]

Arguments in favour of genetic interventions

Below, I shall discuss the following three arguments in favour of genetic interventions: they may be used (1) to cure diseases, (2) to prevent diseases, and (3) to meet the needs and wants of couples and parents.

Curing disease

The best argument in favour of genetic interventions in medicine would no doubt be if these could be used to actually *cure* diseases, or at least to significantly reduce the symptoms.

Clearly, a *working* procedure of S-GT could easily be supported in this way in cases where a sick person would be relieved of his or her health-problem as an effect of the procedure. Imagine, for example, safe S-GT that would enable people with various types of cancer to get rid of this disease, or at least to slow its progression or to reduce its undesirable effects. This would surely be a cure in the ordinary and highly valued sense of the word: a sick person goes through a process which makes him or her less sick.

However, in many cases of genetic diseases, when the symptoms start to appear, the possibility of successful intervention already lies in the past. In many cases, therefore, S-GT would have to be undertaken before the person in question has turned sick.[7] Moreover, many genetic diseases are founded very early in life and would therefore need GL-GT in order to be stopped, a procedure performed in the very beginning of or even before the start of fetal development. In both of these cases, since there is no sick patient that is being treated, it is quite hard to speak of any curing being accomplished.

In the case of GP, to speak of curing becomes even more strange (although some medical specialists seem to endorse such peculiar usage[8]). Here, no changing of a malfunctioning bodily process is involved and, consequently, no sick individual can be cured by GP.

Preventing disease

Might we do better by looking at genetic interventions as *preventive* measures? In that case, the fact that procedures are undertaken before any symptoms have appeared is no objection, rather, it is the very *point*. However, at the same time, the concept of medical prevention is notoriously unclear. We can distinguish between two rough and rather different senses, individual and statistical.

In the case of successful *individual* prevention, someone stays healthy due to the preventive undertaking. For example, successful prevention of cancer and cardiac problems by health-information works in this way. People stay healthy since they quit smoking, exercise more, eat better food etc. as an effect of the information. Clearly, this concept is also applicable to a working procedure of S-GT which prevents the outbreak of some disease in a person.

In contrast, GP is clearly unable to accomplish any prevention in this sense, since GP works through the exchanging of one possible future individual for another one. Thus, we are unable to say about a healthy child born as a result of GP that *this* child has stayed healthy thanks to the GP. For had the GP not been undertaken, *this* child would not have been sick (since it then would never have existed), but *another* one which, in turn, in fact never exists due to the fact that GP in fact *has* been used.

Regarding GL-GT, the following line of thought might be tempting: GL-GT means that the genetic modification is undertaken very early, maybe even before the affected individual exists (if the modified genome resides in the gametes of its parents, grand parents etc.). However, it is still the case that there is *a specific individual* (already existing or one that will exist in the future) which is in this way helped to stay healthy. This individual would have got sick, had the GL-GT not been undertaken. For example, if the genome of an early embryo is modified so that the gene for Huntington's disease is taken out or "blocked", the resulting born person has been helped to stay healthy. Had the GL-GT not been undertaken this person would have become sick with Huntington's disease, and the same goes for a certain percentage of this person's offspring.[9]

There are good reasons to resist this line of thought, however. Due to the technical procedures involved in any presently imaginable process of GL-GT, there will be as much of an exchange of individuals involved as in the case of GP. In order to demonstrate, let us look at how such a process of GL-GT would presumably proceed.[10]

Presently, there are two techniques which may be developed into a working procedure of GL-GT. The first one is the "reprogramming" of the genome of an adult somatic cell back to its initial embryonic state made so famous by the "cloned" sheep Dolly. Since precise genetic modification is much easier to achieve on somatic cells (which, unlike germ-line cells, may be laboratory cultured without limit and tampered with until the desired result is achieved), the "Dolly-procedure" may be used for transplanting the nucleus of such a modified cell into an oocyte (emptied of its own nucleus) which is then reprogrammed into an embryo. Although not yet applied to human beings, present scientific opinion seems to be that such a procedure offers one of the most promising prospects for achieving reliable GL-GT.[11]

It is easy to see how, with such a procedure, it becomes impossible to say that the resulting individual has been helped to stay healthy. For, had the procedure not been undertaken, *this* individual would obviously never have existed. True, had the couple in question procreated in the ordinary way, the result might have been a child suffering from a serious genetic disease. However, *that* child would certainly not have been the *same* child as the healthy one resulting from the procedure just described (apart from the peculiarity of "cloning" itself, it would most probably not even spring from the same oocyte). This line of GL-GT therefore seems to involve as much preselection of possible future individuals as ordinary GP.

The other technique is an even more recent development in cell-biology, enabling successful continuous culturing (or "proliferation") of embryonic "stem-cells" from the blastocyst stage of fetal development. Such cells may therefore be reliably genetically modified just like somatic cells and then injected into a blastocyst, causing effects also in the germ-line. Again, such a procedure has not yet been applied to human beings, but is well-known from the genetic modification of mice since the early 1980's.[12] Moreover, research is presently being done on expanding the possibilities for culturing even further back to the very earliest of human development—the germ-line cells forming the basis for every cell in our bodies.[13]

In this case, no "cloning" is involved. However, the procedure presupposes the use of IVF so that access to embryos is secured. Without going into detail about what this involves, it seems safe to say that the way procreation proceeds in such a setting makes it highly unlikely that a resulting child would be the same as the one that would have resulted had the couple in question chosen to procreate in the ordinary way. Again, therefore, we have a situation where we cannot say that a healthy individual existing as a result of GL-GT has been helped by this procedure to stay healthy. Had the procedure not been used, *this* individual would never have existed, but *another* individual who possibly would have been affected by some genetic disease.

Perhaps, then, a more generous concept of prevention will do the trick? A first step in this direction is to substitute "helped to stay healthy" for "saved from harm." This manoeuvre facilitates that we may say that a possible future child may be saved from harm by having its very existence prevented in a case where this existence would have been worse for this child than not coming into being in the first place.[14] At the same time, however, it must be stressed that the range of applicability of this reasoning very much depends on what basic theory regarding what makes life more or less worth living is accepted. Theories about this which put the emphasis on subjective well-being are probably not potent of making the "saving from harm"-argument applicable in other than the most extreme and comparably rare genetic diseases, such as Tay-Sachs, Krabbe and Werdig-Hoffman. Thus, the argument will not work for common genetic disorders such as Cystic fibrosis or Sickle-cell anemia, unless a theory of the value of life which locates this value in some factor external to the individual's own perception and evaluation of his or her own life is accepted.[15] Moreover, to the extent that this line of reasoning is applicable, the "saved from harm"-argument seems to work equally well for GP and GL-GT.

This takes us to the concept of *statistic* prevention, where the scope is broadened from focusing merely on help for *particular* individuals. In addition, we now consider also comparisons of well-being between different possible future individuals, so that a reduced statistical incidence of disease is counted as a preventive effect even if no one is saved from harm by this reduction. In effect, something is gained by substituting for a possible future child who would have suffered from a disease, *another* possible future child who is healthy. Although the affected child would have had a life worth living, the unaffected child's life is presumably *more* worth living.

It would presumably go against common usage to *call* such an exchange *prevention* (since no one is saved from anything harmful). However, this does not rule out that a *morally relevant benefit* is achieved! Indeed, this seems to be as much a benefit as when teenagers postpone their parenthood until they are more mature and stable so that their later children get better chances in life. Since this line of reasoning presupposes that impersonal increases of well-being are desirable although no one in particular is benefited, it needs to be underpinned by a utilitarian-style ethical framework.[16] Again, we may also note that the justification apparently works equally well for both GP and GL-GT.

Caring for couples and parents

In many cases, genetic interventions are being motivated from a desire to meet the wants and needs of couples at risk for having children with genetic diseases. In as much as the intervention works, both (S- and GL-) GT and GP apparently can be motivated in this way. In all successful cases, the result is a healthy child rather than a sick one. However, there are also some differences worth noting.

First, while GL-GT and GP secures a healthy child from the very start, S-GT works by intervening in a later stage, after a pregnancy has been embarked upon. This is clearly a drawback since the pregnancy will be entangled with worry and anxiety until it has been established that the S-GT was successful. Moreover, in many cases, S-GT will have to involve intra-uterine procedures, meaning that the woman has to be subjected to invasive methods bringing risks for bodily harm to herself as well as miscarriage. Finally, as mentioned earlier, in many cases of genetic disease S-GT will not be able to help since it intervenes too late.

Secondly, GP may turn out to be more effective in meeting the wants of couples than any GT. This is, of course, an empirical question for the future to straighten out. However, since GP has a considerable head start on GT (it is already clinically applied with moderately successful results) and does not involve the complex task of achieving precise changes of the genome, there may be some reason to believe that GT will remain a secondary option also when the procedures have been made safe and reliable.

It should be noted, however, that not all couples and prospective parents *can* be helped by GP. In cases of where a disease is *dominantly* inherited (one copy of the gene is enough for becoming sick) and an individual carries two copies of the gene, all embryos springing from this person's gametes will be affected. Many dominantly inherited diseases are so-called *late onset*, i.e. the symptoms appear after adolescence, thus making the individual perfectly capable of procreating.

For those where GP *could* help, perhaps GL-GT would still be preferable from the couples point of view? One reason for believing this might be that they can be expected to feel uneasy about the obvious selection of individuals being carried out in GP (at least in the form of PGD). However, as was seen above, the presupposition that this constitutes a difference to GL-GT is in fact a chimera.

Arguments against genetic interventions

Let me now turn to the standard objections to GP and GT. Three arguments will be considered: that genetic interventions are unnatural, that they give too much power to experts, and that they bring risks of a new era of eugenics.

Against Nature

The claim that GT/GP is unnatural may be interpreted in roughly three main ways. According to the first, being natural is an explicitly normative/evaluative concept.[17] The argument then is that GT/GP is wrong since it is not in accordance with the *proper* order of nature (though it may very well be in accordance with the *actual* order of nature described by science). As far as I can see, this line of interpretation makes the argument disappear and turn into the very claim it purports to support: the line of thought becomes tautologous i. e. that there is something wrong with GT/GP since there is something wrong with it. *Why* is it wrong? *What* makes the difference between an *im*proper and a proper order of nature? Such questions remain to be answered, but cannot be answered by again invoking the idea of a proper natural order. It remains an open question, then, to what extent GT and GP is or is not equally wrong (including not wrong at all) according to this interpretation of the objection.

If "natural" is used in a descriptive sense we can note that both GT and GP are perfectly in accordance with the way in which nature works; where they not, they would not be feasible in the first place. Moreover, nature itself performs both of the functions attainable through GT and GP. It is a well-known fact within reproductive medicine that nature selects embryos and gametes; presumably, our biological apparatus also has some influence on our choices of partners. Nature also produces genetic changes on both the somatic and the germ-line level.

This brings us to the idea that genetic interventions change "the course of nature"—they make things different than they would otherwise have been. This is true, of course, but it is hard to see that this should constitute any *objection* since all human activities change the course of nature in this sense. Moreover, this fact seems to hold equally for GP and GT.

Too much power for experts

This objection has been most forcefully put forward by feminist critics of, for example, assisted procreation, prenatal diagnosis and PGD,[18] and there is certainly something to it. The more technical the setting of procreation becomes, the higher the risk that our choices are being (intentionally or unintentionally) manipulated by the experts who perform the various procedures involved. Moreover, the increased technical setting also means that society may feel more tempted to demand certain choices to be made by people, since these choices are effected in a laboratory rather than inside the body of a person.

This objection works equally well for GP and GT, in as much as they involve the degree of technicality assumed (certain kinds of GP need not, as we saw above). However, the objection does not speak against GP or GT *as such*, but rather against certain ways of organising and performing such procedures. It seems clear that what is needed is a clinical as well as societal setting where procreative autonomy is highly safeguarded. It is a virtue of the feminist criticism to have made this urgent need more salient.[19]

Risks for eugenics

To choose one's children on genetic grounds or to deliberately engineer their genetic make-up is, it has been claimed, a form of eugenics relevantly similar to that of Nazi-Germany or the policies of compulsory sterilisation practised throughout the West during the 20th century.[20] I shall not go deeply into the adequacy of this analogy,[21] but will content myself with pointing out that mere applicability of the word "eugenics" constitutes no objection as such. What is needed for an objection is reason to believe that genetic interventions would recreate some of those features which made the old eugenic policies morally objectionable. Let me therefore distinguish between three senses or aspects of the concept of eugenics.

The first is to focus on the selection of *characteristics* of children. Obviously, both GT and GP involve such selection. But we also select our children's characteristics when we choose a partner from the point of view of looks, personality, social status etc., when we contribute to the forming of children's personalities through upbringing, education etc., and, not least, when we safeguard our children's health through good environment, nutrition and health care.

How about eugenics as the selection of *individuals* then? This aspect is obviously not present in the case of S-GT, since the intervention there is made on a particular individual. However, in the case of GP, such selection is the very core of what is being done. As was argued above, this is actually also the case with GL-GT.

It might be suggested that, although both GP and GL-GT involve the selection of (possible future) individuals, the selection in GP is much more *salient*.[22] Consider, for example, GP achieved through PGD, where one or two early embryos out of-say-ten present in the laboratory are selected for transfer into a woman's uterus. However, on reflection, this impression seems mainly to be a function of lack of knowledge of how GL-GT in fact would work. Consider, for example, the selection of one genetically modified somatic cell-nucleus out of, say, 2000 available in the laboratory, which is then transplanted into one of 10 available (enucleated) oocytes (followed by the "Dolly-style" reactivating procedure transforming this oocyte into an early embryo).

In any case, it is hard to see that the fact that they involve selection of individuals constitutes any objection *as such* to GP and GL-GT. If it did, it would be an equally strong objection against *all* family-planning. When a teenager chooses to postpone parenthood, the child he or she will have in, say, ten years will evidently not be the same child as the one he or she would have had, had he/she instead chosen to have children immediately. Had my mother chosen to have children with someone else than my father, perhaps they would have had a son who would now have been of my age, but he would certainly not have been *me*. Actually, when people in this way plan the timing of family-formation in their lives, as well as choose partner, with the expected child's well-being in mind, they are generally regarded as *especially* morally responsible. Why not say the same regarding the use of GP and GL-GT?

In fact, when people allude to eugenics in debates about genetics, what they mainly express is a fear of systematic pressure on, or outright coercion of, people to have children living up to some more or less clearly defined "standard of perfection." Such pressure may come from the state, as was the case with the policies of compulsory sterilisation. However, they may also arise out of heightened expectations regarding what qualities our children are to have resulting from a widespread use of genetic interventions—a process which have been called "backdoor eugenics."[23]

Obviously, such pressures may arise whether or not we consider GP or GT. In the case of S-GT, however, the pressure may seem to be completely acceptable and not very different from the raised expectations that children will not to die from common child-diseases due to the appearance of effective treatments and preventive measures. In contrast, in the case of GP and GL-GT, the situation is different, since these procedures involve choosing *which* children have, not only choosing whether or not one's children are to be healthy or not. Pressures on people to use GP or GL-GT would thus constitute a grave infringement of their procreative autonomy—which children are born would be dictated by the state or the "market" of socio-economic expectations and available techniques.

Obviously, the best defence against such developments is the insistence on people's unconditional legal right to full procreative autonomy. However, *formal* protection of this right is not sufficient. Open coercion is not the only force through which procreative autonomy may be reduced—social processes making the choice of *not* using GP or GL-GT extremely unattractive may have similar effects. In particular, the willingness of the general public to pay for acceptable care and support for disabled children may weaken when the common choice is to avoid having such children through GP or GL-GT. It is therefore important that procreative liberty is upheld as a *real* possibility and not only a formal right. If it is not, procreative autonomy will be radically undermined and we will have a society sharing one crucial feature with past societies employing eugenic policies.

In practice, this means that the common idea of listing conditions which are fit for GP/GL-GT and those that are not, or to make some general distinction between therapy and "enhancement" for the same purpose, is actually utterly suspect. What we get is a publicly sanctioned ideology regarding what kind of people should exist; it is allright to have brown eyes, but not allright to have a cardiac condition or an IQ below 70, for example. This obviously introduces exactly the kind of pressure making up the essence of eugenic policies of the past.[24] Another important implication is that the ethical quality of the clinical application of GP and GL-GT is dependent on the policies pursued in society at large. The ethical reflection of clinicians in these fields therefore needs to take such factors into account.[25]

Concluding remarks: Why not germ-line gene therapy?

Let me sum up the points made so far. From an ethical point of view, the difference between, on the one hand, GP and GL-GT and, on the other, S-GT is much greater than that between GP and GT in general. GP and GL-GT also actualise more hard ethical issues than does S-GT. On the other hand, the applicability of S-GT is limited since many genetic conditions are founded so early in human development.

Since GP is actually clinically applied today in many countries, how could the common resistance to GL-GT be motivated? Both strategies involve intervention on the germ-line level. Furthermore, there are cases where GP is unable to help but where GL-GT could be so able.

Presumably, the standard-answer would refer to the risks for the offspring associated with GL-GT. Now, as was seen above, the risk that the offspring is actually *harmed* in this way is in fact much less than is commonly assumed (since GL-GT, just like GP, involves an interchange of different possible future people). This does not rule out that the risks may involve an (unintentional) increase of harmful *conditions*. However, if this is to be taken to speak against GL-GT, utilitarian ways of thinking taking *im*personal changes of well-being into account have to be accepted.

Of course, there is reason for great *caution* when introducing GL-GT. However, there is no reason to limit such caution to methods which are explicitly *intended* to effect genetic changes. Although the *intention* in GP is not to change the genome, the techniques used in, for example, PGD may nevertheless effect such changes.[26] Apparently, authorities have been aware of this fact when giving the green light for PGD. Were they wrong to do so? Moreover, the caution must also involve a balancing of risks against *possible benefits* in terms of chances to reduce harmful genetic conditions compared to alternative means for achieving this (GP or environmental intervention). I have given some reason above for believing that such balancing may turn out to speak in favour of GP in relation to GL-GT in cases where both strategies are applicable.[27]

Notes

1. See Walters et. al., 1997, and Friedmann, 1997.
2. Comprehensible overviews of the present state of GT, as well as future prospects and hopes are provided in Walters et. al., 1997, and a special report consisting of Blaese, 1997, Felgner, 1997, Friedmann, 1997, Ho, et. al., 1997, and Mirsky, et. al., 1997.
3. See, for example, Munthe, 1996a.
4. It should be noted, though, that some people indeed *would*. Clinical geneticists have told me about several cases where couples have broken up their marriage or partnership when they have been informed about the risk of their possible children inheriting diseases.
5. See, for example, Chadwick, 1987.
6. For overviews of such methods, see Handyside, 1996 and Verlinsky et. al., 1997. In Munthe, 1999c, I address ethical and political issues actualised by these methods as well as possible future ones arising from them.
7. This presupposes that being the carrier of a gene which poses a threat to one's future health is not the same as being affected by a disease. Since many genes predisposing for disease do not guarantee future sickness, there appear to be good reasons for such usage.

8. In a set of ethical guidelines published by the American Fertility Society, PGD is spoken of as a way of "*correcting* serious and life-threatening genetic defects". See Ethics Committee of the American Fertility Society, 1994, p. 91S. The italics have been added by me.
9. Harris, 1993, Walters et.al., 1997, pp. 80–81, 85. See also Nikolaus Knoeppfler's contribution to the present volume.
10. More or less the same point, but in relation to possible applications of genetic technologies within sports, is made in Munthe, 1999a.
11. "Adult Cloning Marches On", Ashworth et.al., 1998, Mirsky et.al., 1997, Signer et.al., 1998, Solter, 1998, Wakayama et.al., 1998, Wilmut et.al., 1997.
12. Gearhart, 1998, Marshall, 1998, Thomson et.al., 1998.
13. Handyside, 1996.
14. Cf. Harris, 1993.
15. Cf. Munthe, 1996a, chapter 3, and Munthe, 1999c.
16. This introduces other considerations as well, of course. These, as well as the argument sketched here, are pursued much more thoroughly in Munthe, 1998 and 1999c.
17. This idea, of course, is the common one in religious ethics where "nature" and "natural law" often refers to "(God's ideas about) how nature *should* be".
18. See, for example, Arditti et.al., 1989, Bonnicksen, 1992, Corea, 1988, Hubbard, 1990, Hubbard et.al., 1993, Katz Rothman, 1992, Knoppers et.al., 1993, Lippman, 1991 and Overall, 1987.
19. In Munthe, 1999c, I discuss at length what such safeguarding of procreative autonomy implies in terms of requirements on and organisation of the practice of GP.
20. Bonnicksen, 1992, Ewing, 1988, Knoppers et.al., 1993, Krimsky et.al., 1995, Testart, 1995, Wertz, 1992.
21. I discuss it thoroughly in Munthe, 1999c.
22. I have encountered this line of thought in my discussions with Swedish health care personnel involved in PGD. See Munthe, 1999c.
23. Duster, 1990.
24. Cf. Munthe, 1996b, 1999b, and 1999c.
25. Cf. Munthe, 1996a, and Munthe et.al., 1998.
26. The future of the approximately 160 children born after PGD (see Verlinsky et.al. 1998), as well as their children, will hopefully eventually make us wiser on this point.
27. I wish to thank Kees Dekker, Nikolaus Knoeppfler, Jan Wahlström and Lars Ährlund-Richter for helpful discussions and/or scientific guidance.

Bibliography

"Adult Cloning Marches On" anonymous editorial, Nature 394, p. 303.

Arditti, R., Klein, R. D., Minden, S. (eds.), 1989. Test Tube Women: What Future for Womanhood? Pandora Press: London.

Ashworth, D., Bishop, M., Campbell, K., Colman, A., Kind, A., Schnieke, A., Blott, S., Griffin, H., Haley, C., McWhir, J., Wilmut, I., 1998. "DNA Microsatellite Analysis of Dolly." Nature 394, p. 329.

Blaese, R. M., 1997. "Gene Therapy for Cancer." Scientific American 276, 6, pp. 111–115.

Bonnicksen, A., 1992. "Genetic Diagnosis of Human Embryos." In: "Genetic Grammar." Special supplement. Hastings Center Report 22, 4, S5–S11.

Chadwick, R. F., 1987. "The Perfect Baby: Introduction." In: Chadwick R. F. (ed.). Ethics, Reproduction and Genetic Control. Routledge: London, New York.

Corea, G., 1988. The Mother Machine. Reproductive Technologies from Artificial Insemination to Artificial Wombs. The Women's Press: London.

Duster, T., 1990. Backdoor to Eugenics. Routledge: London, New York.

Ethics Committee of the American Fertility Society, 1994. "Ethical Considerations of Assisted Reproductive Technologies." Fertility and Sterility 62, 5, supplement 1.

Ewing, C. M., 1988. "Tailored Genes: IVF, Genetic Engineering and Eugenics." Reproductive and Genetic Engineering 1, 1, pp. 31–40.

Felgner, P. L., 1997. "Nonviral Strategies for Gene Therapy." Scientific American 276, 6, pp. 102–106.

Friedmann, T., 1997. "Overcoming Obstacles to Gene Therapy." Scientific American 276, 6, pp. 96–101.

Gearhart, J., 1998. "New Potential for Human Embryonic Stem Cells." Science 282, pp. 1061–1062.

Handyside, A., 1996. "Preimplantation Genetic Diagnosis Today." Human Reproduction, 11, supplement 1, pp. 139–151.

Harris, J., 1993. "Is Gene Therapy a Form of Eugenics?" Bioethics 7, 2–3, pp. 178–187.

Ho, D. O., Sapolsky, R. M., 1997. "Gene Therapy for the Nervous System." Scientific American 276, 6, pp. 116–120.

Hubbard, R., 1990. The Politics of Women's Biology. Rutgers University Press: New Brunswick.

Hubbard, R., Wald, E., 1993. Exploding the Gene Myth: How Genetic Information is Produced and Manipulated by Scientists, Physicians, Employers, Insurance Companies, Educators, and Law Enforcers. Beacon Press: Boston.

Katz Rothman, B., 1992. "Not All that Glitter is Gold." In: "Genetic Grammar." Special Supplement. Hastings Center Report 22, 4, S11–S15.

Knoppers, B., Le Bris, S., 1993. "Reproductive Genetics: Canadian and European Perspectives." Fetal Diagnosis and Therapy 8, supplement 1, pp. 189–201.

Krimsky, S., Hubbard, R., 1995. "The Business of Research." Hastings Center Report 25, 1, pp. 41–43.

Lippman, A., 1991. "Prenatal Genetic Testing and Screening: Constructing Needs and Reinforcing Inequities." Journal of Law and Medicine 17, pp. 15–50.

Marshall, E., 1998. "A Versatile Cell Line Raises Scientific Hopes, Legal Questions." Science 282, pp. 1014–1015.

Mirsky, S., Rennie, J., 1997. "What Cloning Means for Gene Therapy." Scientific American 276, 6, pp. 122–123.

Munthe, C., 1996a. The Moral Roots of Prenatal Diagnosis. Studies in Research Ethics no. 7. Centre for Research Ethics: Göteborg.

Munthe, C., 1996b, "Abortion: From Ethics to Politics." EAGO Newsletter 2, 2, pp. 25–28.

Munthe, C., 1998. "On Choosing Children." In: Kampits P., Kokai K., Weiberg A. (eds.). Applied Ethics. Papers of the 21st International Wittgenstein Symposium. Volume VI (2). Austrian Ludwig Wittgenstein Society: Kirchberg am Wechsel.

Munthe, C., 1999a. "Selected Champions. Making Winners in the Age of Genetic Technology." In: Tamburrini C et.al. (eds.), 1999. Sports and Values. Routledge: London (forthcoming).

Munthe, C., 1999b. "Testing for Personality Traits: Four Lessons from Prenatal Diagnosis." In: Welin, S. (ed.), 1999. Genetics and Behaviour. Studies in Research Ethics no. 8. Centre for Research Ethics: Göteborg (forthcoming).

Munthe, C., 1999c. Pure Selection. The Ethics of Preimplantation Genetic Diagnosis and Choosing Children without Abortion (unpublished manuscript).

Munthe, C., Wahlström, J., Welin, S., 1998. "Fosterdiagnostikens moraliska rötter. Goda handikappomsorger avgörande för den etiska kvaliteten." Läkartidningen 95, 8, pp. 750–753.

Overall, C., 1987. Ethics and Human Reproduction: A Feminist Analysis. Allen & Unwin: Winchester, Maryland.

Signer, E. N., Dubrova, Y. E., Jeffreys, A. J., Wilde, C., Finch, L. M. P., Wells, M., Peaker, M., 1998. "DNA Fingerprinting Dolly." Nature 394, p. 329.

Solter, D., 1998, "Dolly Is a Clone- and No Longer Alone." Nature 394, p. 315.

Testart, J., 1995. "The New Eugenics and Medicalized Reproduction." Cambridge Quarterly of Health Care Ethics 4, pp. 304–312.

Thomson, J. A., Itskovitz-Eldor, J., Shapiro, S. S., Waknitz, M. A., Swiergiel, J. J., Marshall, V. S., Jones, J. M., 1998. "Embryonic Stem Cell Lines Derived from Human Blastocysts." Science 282, pp. 1145–1147.

Verlinsky, Y., Munné, S., Simpson, J. L., Kuliev, A., Ao, A., Ray, P., Sermon, K., Martin, R., Strom, C., Van Stairteghem, A., Veiga, A., Drury, K., Williams, S., Ginsberg, N., Wilton, L., 1997. "Current Status of Preimplantation Diagnosis." Journal of Assisted Reproduction and Genetics 14, pp. 72–75.

Verlinsky, Y., Kuliev, A., 1998. "Progress in Preimplantation Genetics." Journal of Assisted Reproduction and Genetics 15, 1, pp. 9–11.

Wakayama, T., Perry, A. C. F., Zuccotti, M., Johnson, K. R., Yanagimachi, R., 1998. "Full-term Development of Mice from Enucleated Oocytes Injected with Cumulus Cell Nuclei." Nature 394, pp. 369–374.

Walters, L., Palmer, J. G., 1997. The Ethics of Human Gene Therapy. Oxford University Press: New York, Oxford.

Wertz, D. C., 1992. "Ethical and Legal Implications of the New Genetics: Issues for Discussion." Social Science Medicine 35, 4, pp. 495–505.

Wilmut, I., Schnieke, A. E., McWhir, J., Kind, A. J., Campbell, K. H., 1997. "Viable Offspring Derived from Fetal and Adult Mammalian Cells." Nature 385, pp. 810–813.

Contributors

Malcolm Brenner
Professor
Texas Children's Hospital &
Baylor College of Medicin
6621 Fannin St.
Houston MC3-3320
U.S.A.

Kris Dierickx
Dr.
Centre for Biomedical Ethics and Las
Kapucünen voer 35
B-3000 Leuven
Belgium

Sigrid Graumann
Dr.
Centre for Ethics in the Sciences and Humanities
University Tübingen
Keplerstrasse 17
D-720 74 Tübingen
Germany

Eric Juengst
Associate Professor
Center for Biomedical Ethics
School of Medicine
Case Western Reserve University
Euclid Avenue 10900
Cleveland OH 44106
U.S.A.

Rihito Kimura
Professor
Director of Internat./Asian Bioethics Program
Kennedy Institute of Ethics
Georgetown University
Washington D.C. 20057-212
U.S.A.
(also Department of Human Health Sciences
School of Human Sciences
Waseda University
Tokyo & Tokorozawa
Japan)

Nikolaus Knoepffler
Dr.
Institut Technik-Theology-Naturwissenschaften
Marsstrasse 19
D-80335 Munich
Germany

Karen Lebacqz
Professor
Theological Ethics
Pacific School of Religion
1798 Scenic Avenue
Berkeley CA 94709
U.S.A.

Dietmar Mieth
Professor
Interfaculty Center for Ethics in the Sciences and Humanities
University of Tübingen
D-72074 Tübingen
Germany

Christian Munthe
Associate Professor
Departement of Philosophy
Göteborg University
Box 200
SE-405 30 Göteborg
Sweden

Anders Nordgren
Research Scholar
Department of Public Health and Caring Sciences
(Biomedical Ethics)
Uppsala Science Park
SE-751 85 Uppsala
Sweden
(formerly Director,
Centre for Research Ethics,
Uppsala University)

Edvard Smith
Associate Professor
Center for Biotechnology
Karolinska Institutet
141 57 Stockholm
Sweden

LeRoy Walters
Professor, Director
The Kennedy Institute of Ethics
Georgetown University
Box 571 212
Washington D.C. 200 57-1212
U.S.A.

Charles Weiner | Professor emeritus
(at Massachussetts Institute of Technology)
56 Main Street
Yarmouth Port MA 02675
U.S.A.